Hypercoagulable States and New Anticoagulants

Guest Editors

MARK CROWTHER, MD, MSc, FRCPC
MARCO P. DONADINI, MD

HEMATOLOGY/ONCOLOGY CLINICS OF NORTH AMERICA

www.hemonc.theclinics.com

Consulting Editors
GEORGE P. CANELLOS, MD
NANCY BERLINER, MD

August 2010 • Volume 24 • Number 4

SAUNDERS an imprint of ELSEVIER, Inc.

W.B. SAUNDERS COMPANY
A Division of Elsevier Inc.

1600 John F. Kennedy Blvd. ● Suite 1800 ● Philadelphia, PA 19103-2899

http://www.theclinics.com

HEMATOLOGY/ONCOLOGY CLINICS OF NORTH AMERICA Volume 24, Number 4
August 2010 ISSN 0889-8588, ISBN 13: 978-1-4377-2529-2

Editor: Kerry Holland

Hematology/Oncology Clinics (ISSN 0889-8588) is published bimonthly by Elsevier Inc., 360 Park Avenue South, New York, NY 10010-1710. Months of issue are February, April, June, August, October, and December. Business and Editorial Offices: 1600 John F. Kennedy Blvd., Ste. 1800, Philadelphia, PA 19103–2899. Customer Service Office: 3251 Riverport Lane, Maryland Heights, MO 63043. Periodicals postage paid at New York, NY and at additional mailing offices. Subscription prices are $306.00 per year (domestic individuals), $483.00 per year (domestic institutions), $152.00 per year (domestic students/residents), $347.00 per year (Canadian individuals), $591.00 per year (Canadian institutions) $413.00 per year (international individuals), $591.00 per year (international institutions), and $206.00 per year (international and Canadian students/residents). International air speed delivery is included in all *Clinics* subscription prices. All prices are subject to change without notice. **POSTMASTER:** Send address changes to *Hematology/Oncology Clinics of North America*, Elsevier Health Sciences Division, Subscription Customer Service, 3251 Riverport Lane, Maryland Heights, MO 63043. Customer Service (orders, claims, online, change of address): Elsevier Health Sciences Division, Subscription Customer Service, 3251 Riverport Lane, Maryland Heights, MO 63043. Tel: 1-800-654-2452 (U.S. and Canada); 314-447-8871 (outside U.S. and Canada). Fax: 314-447-8029. E-mail: journalscustomerservice-usa@elsevier.com (for print support); journalsonlinesupport-usa@elsevier.com (for online support).

Reprints. For copies of 100 or more, of articles in this publication, please contact the Commercial Reprints Department, Elsevier Inc., 360 Park Avenue South, New York, New York 10010-1710; Tel.: 212-633-3813, Fax: 212-462-1935, E-mail: reprints@elsevier.com.

Hematology/Oncology Clinics of North America is covered in *MEDLINE/PubMed (Index Medicus), EMBASE/Excerpta Medica, and BIOSIS.*

Printed and bound by CPI Group (UK) Ltd, Croydon, CR0 4YY

Transferred to Digital Print 2011

Contributors

CONSULTING EDITORS

GEORGE P. CANELLOS, MD
William Rosenberg Professor of Medicine, Department of Medical Oncology, Dana-Farber Cancer Institute, Boston, Massachusetts

NANCY BERLINER, MD
Chief, Division of Hematology, Brigham and Women's Hospital; Professor of Medicine, Harvard Medical School, Boston, Massachusetts

GUEST EDITORS

MARK CROWTHER, MD, MSc, FRCPC
Professor and Chair, Division of Hematology and Thromboembolism, St Joseph's Hospital, McMaster University, Hamilton, Ontario, Canada

MARCO P. DONADINI, MD
Formerly, Research Fellow, Division of Hematology and Thromboembolism, St Joseph's Hospital, McMaster University, Hamilton, Ontario, Canada; Currently, Division of Internal Medicine 1, University of Insubria, Circolo Hospital, Varese, Italy

AUTHORS

WALTER AGENO, MD
Associate Professor of Medicine, Department of Clinical Medicine, Research Center on Thromboembolic Disorders and Antithrombotic Therapies, University of Insubria, Circolo Hospital, Varese, Italy

JACK E. ANSELL, MD
Chairman, Department of Medicine, Lenox Hill Hospital, New York, New York

LORENA APPIO, MD
Department of Clinical Medicine, Research Center on Thromboembolic Disorders and Antithrombotic Therapies, University of Insubria, Varese, Italy

GAURI BADHWAR, DO
Department of Medicine, Lenox Hill Hospital, New York, New York

LORENZA BRIVIO, MD
Department of Clinical Medicine, Research Center on Thromboembolic Disorders and Antithrombotic Therapies, University of Insubria, Varese, Italy

HARRY R. BÜLLER, MD
Department of Vascular Medicine, Academic Medical Center Amsterdam, Amsterdam, The Netherlands

DEBORAH J. COOK, MD
Departments of Medicine and Clinical Epidemiology and Biostatistics, McMaster University, Hamilton, Ontario, Canada

MARK CROWTHER, MD, MSc, FRCPC
Professor and Chair, Division of Hematology and Thromboembolism, St Joseph's Hospital, McMaster University, Hamilton, Ontario, Canada

FRANCESCO DENTALI, MD
Department of Clinical Medicine, Research Center on Thromboembolic Disorders and Antithrombotic Therapies, University of Insubria, Varese, Italy

MARCO P. DONADINI, MD
Formerly, Research Fellow, Division of Hematology and Thromboembolism, St Joseph's Hospital, McMaster University, Hamilton, Ontario, Canada; Currently, Division of Internal Medicine 1, University of Insubria, Circolo Hospital, Varese, Italy

JAMES D. DOUKETIS, MD, FRCP(C)
Department of Medicine, St Joseph's Healthcare Hamilton, McMaster University, Hamilton, Ontario, Canada

DAVID GARCIA, MD
Associate Professor, Division of Hematology and Oncology, Department of Internal Medicine, University of New Mexico School of Medicine, Albuquerque, New Mexico

CATHERINE J. LEE, MD
Department of Medicine, Lenox Hill Hospital, New York, New York

ERICA ROMUALDI, MD
Resident in Internal Medicine, Department of Clinical Medicine, Research Center on Thromboembolic Disorders and Antithrombotic Therapies, University of Insubria, Circolo Hospital, Varese, Italy

ALESSANDRO SQUIZZATO, MD, PhD
Department of Clinical Medicine, Research Center on Thromboembolic Disorders and Antithrombotic Therapies, University of Insubria, Varese, Italy

JOANNA UENG, MD
Department of Medicine, St Joseph's Healthcare Hamilton, McMaster University, Hamilton, Ontario, Canada

FREDERIEK F. VAN DOORMAAL, MD
Department of Vascular Medicine, Academic Medical Center Amsterdam, Amsterdam, The Netherlands

THEODORE E. WARKENTIN, MD
Departments of Pathology and Molecular Medicine, Department of Medicine, Michael G. DeGroote School of Medicine, McMaster University; Transfusion Medicine, Hamilton Regional Laboratory Medicine Program; Service of Clinical Hematology, Hamilton Health Sciences, Hamilton General Hospital, Hamilton, Ontario, Canada

JOHN WINTERS, MD
Resident, Department of Internal Medicine, University of New Mexico School of Medicine, Albuquerque, New Mexico

DANIEL M. WITT, PharmD, FCCP, BCPS, CACP
Senior Manager, Clinical Pharmacy Services and Research, Department of Pharmacy, Kaiser Permanente Colorado, Aurora, Colorado

Contents

**Antiphospholipid Syndrome: A Challenging Hypercoagulable State
with Systemic Manifestations**   **669**

Marco P. Donadini and Mark Crowther

> Antiphospholipid syndrome (APS) is a systemic disease that causes venous and arterial thrombosis in virtually any organ and is responsible for fetal losses and pregnancy disorders. Previously, APS was thought to be present mainly in patients with systemic lupus erythematosus. The spectrum of clinical manifestations is wide, because the thrombotic process may involve arterial and venous vessels of any size in any organ. At present, there is no evidence to support or refute specific treatment strategies for primary prophylaxis of thrombosis.

Pulmonary Embolism in Medical-Surgical Critically Ill Patients   **677**

Deborah J. Cook and Marco P. Donadini

> Pulmonary embolism (PE) is the most dangerous complication of venous thrombosis. Objectively confirmed PE is a potentially life-threatening complication of critical illness. In medical-surgical critically ill patients, signs and symptoms are nonspecific, the clinical pretest probability may be low, and diagnostic tests may not be done or may yield ambiguous results. Therefore, PE is often undiagnosed and untreated; autopsy findings indicate that PE is common in intensive care unit (ICU) decedents. PE may delay weaning from mechanical ventilation, increase the length of stay in ICU and hospital, and increase the risk of death. More research is needed on PE in medical-surgical ICU patients including issues on the epidemiologic aspects of PE (including risk factors and attributable morbidity and mortality) and treatment of PE (including pharmacologic and nonpharmacologic approaches, determinants of treatment variation, and predictors of PE outcome adjusted for treatment).

**Prevention and Treatment of Hormone-Associated Venous Thromboembolism:
A Patient Management Approach**   **683**

Joanna Ueng and James D. Douketis

> Given the known increased risk of venous thromboembolism (VTE) associated with both oral contraceptive (OC) use and hormone replacement therapy (HRT), it is important to address questions about the prevention and management of hormone-associated VTE. Specifically, the objectives of this article are as follows: (1) to provide suggested clinical management approaches for the primary and secondary prevention of VTE for women with thrombophilia; (2) to provide suggested clinical management

a convenient route of administration, can be given in fixed doses, and do not require coagulation monitoring. Favorable results of clinical trials support their potential to change current practice. Translation into daily clinical practice may take some time; clinical studies over the next months and years will reveal the impact of rivaroxaban and other compounds in development. The aim of this review is to provide an overview of the more advanced oral, direct factor Xa inhibitors and to briefly describe the results of the completed studies.

Catherine J. Lee, Gauri Badhwar, and Jack E. Ansell

Direct oral factor IIa inhibitors represent a new class of anticoagulants for the prevention and treatment of venous and selected arterial thromboembolisms. Dabigatran etexilate is the most studied and promising of the oral direct thrombin inhibitors. Preclinical and early-phase clinical studies show it to have a predictable and reliable pharmacokinetic and pharmacodynamic profile, whereas advanced phase 3 trials prove it to be noninferior to traditional anticoagulants in selective conditions for the prevention and treatment of venous and arterial thromboembolism. Other advantages of this drug, including a lack of interaction with cytochrome P450 enzymes or with food and drugs, rapid onset of action, good safety profile, lack of need for routine monitoring, broad therapeutic window, and fixed-dose administration, make this a competitive oral anticoagulant.

Theodore E. Warkentin

Heparin-induced thrombocytopenia (HIT) is an immune-mediated adverse drug effect characterized by platelet activation, hypercoagulability, and increased risk of thrombosis, both venous and arterial. A diagnosis of HIT usually signifies that heparin products, including unfractionated and low-molecular-weight heparin, are contraindicated. Although it is uncertain whether heparin continuation really worsens clinical outcomes, it is clear that vitamin K antagonists such as warfarin do worsen outcomes, as they promote microvascular thrombosis, with the potential for limb amputation (venous limb gangrene). Thus, alternative nonheparin anticoagulants are at the forefront of HIT therapy. This review proposes that alternative anticoagulants (danaparoid, fondaparinux) that share certain properties of heparin—namely its irreversible antithrombin-mediated inhibition of factor Xa—and that have relatively long half-lives, have several advantages in the therapy for HIT over short-acting agents that inhibit thrombin directly (recombinant hirudin, argatroban, and bivalirudin).

Frederiek F. van Doormaal and Harry R. Büller

The bi-directional association between cancer and the coagulation system has been known for almost 2 centuries. During the past 2 decades research has focused on the precise mechanisms through which cancer cells are able to induce a hypercoagulable state and how this leads to an environment favorable for cancer growth. Furthermore, the potential inhibitory effect of anticoagulant drugs on cancer progression has been explored. This article discusses these two aspects of the association.

RELATED INTEREST

Clinics in Laboratory Medicine, June 2009 (Vol. 29, No. 2)
Hemostasis and Coagulation
Henry M. Rinder, MD, *Guest Editor*

THE CLINICS ARE NOW AVAILABLE ONLINE!

Access your subscription at:
www.theclinics.com

Preface

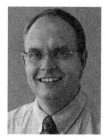 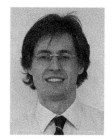

Mark Crowther, MD, MSc, FRCPC   Marco P. Donadini, MD
Guest Editors

In this issue of *Hematology/Oncology Clinics of North America*, the reader will find interesting insights into pathophysiologic conditions that predict hypercoagulability and an update on new anticogulant drugs. As Guest Editors, we chose to present a series of contemporary topics on these 2 themes, inviting well-recognized experts to contribute. We would like to thank each author for their collaboration and the Editors for their guidance.

The first section of this issue is dedicated to hypercoagulable states. It begins with a typical example of a challenging systemic condition involving both venous and arterial thrombosis: the antiphospholipid syndrome. The next article deals with venous thromboembolism (VTE), particularly pulmonary embolism, in critically ill patients. The prevention and treatment of hormone-associated VTE are discussed in the following article, using an evidence-based approach. Another example of systemic activation of coagulation is represented by cancer; this is explored comprehensively with specific regard to its relationship with thrombosis. Finally, insight is provided into the most novel risk factors for VTE, such as endocrine disorders and Jak-2 mutation.

The second part of this issue provides an update on the new anticoagulant drugs, the oral factor-Xa and factor-IIa inhibitors. These drugs will significantly change the management of venous and arterial thromboembolism. This issue also provides special consideration to optimal use of current anticoagulants. Finally, the reader will find up-to-date reviews of the treatment of heparin-induced thrombocytopenia and the relationship between heparin use and survival in cancer patients.

Hematol Oncol Clin N Am 24 (2010) xiii–xiv
doi:10.1016/j.hoc.2010.06.011
0889-8588/10/$ – see front matter © 2010 Elsevier Inc. All rights reserved.

hemonc.theclinics.com

We hope, with this special issue, that we have provided an interesting and up-to-date tool for readers; we wish you enjoyable reading.

Mark Crowther, MD, MSc, FRCPC
Division of Hematology & Thromboembolism
St Joseph's Hospital, McMaster University
50 Charlton Avenue, East, Room L208
Hamilton, ON L8N 4A6, Canada

Marco P. Donadini, MD
Division of Internal Medicine 1
University of Insubria - Circolo Hospital
Viale Borri, Number 57
21100 Varese, Italy

E-mail addresses:
crowthrm@mcmaster.ca (M. Crowther)
collin_dnd@hotmail.com (M.P. Donadini)

Antiphospholipid Syndrome: A Challenging Hypercoagulable State with Systemic Manifestations

Marco P. Donadini, MD, Mark Crowther, MD, MSc, FRCPC*

KEYWORDS

- Antiphospholipid syndrome • aPL-Abs • CAPS • β_2GPI

Antiphospholipid syndrome (APS) is a systemic disease that causes venous and arterial thrombosis in virtually any organ and is responsible for fetal losses and pregnancy disorders.[1] The recognition of APS as an independent nosologic entity is relatively recent, dating back to the late 1980s. Previously, APS was thought to be present mainly in patients with systemic lupus erythematosus (SLE). During the 1970s and 1980s, there were already case reports or small case series describing the association between thrombotic events, fetal loss, and a circulating lupus anticoagulant (LA), without SLE.[2–4] However, it was only in the late 1980s that the existence of a primary APS (ie, in absence of SLE) was postulated.[5,6] An international consensus statement on classification criteria of APS was published in 1999[7] and updated in 2006.[1] Antiphospholipid antibodies (aPL-Abs) constitute a heterogeneous family of autoantibodies directed against proteins that bind to anionic phospholipids and are the basis of the prothrombotic state that characterizes APS.

The spectrum of clinical manifestations is wide, because the thrombotic process may involve arterial and venous vessels of any size in any organ; deep vein thrombosis (DVT) of the lower limbs, pulmonary embolism (PE), stroke or transient ischemic attack (TIA), and myocardial infarction (MI) are some of the most common thrombotic events. Fetal manifestations include early and late fetal loss and premature birth, representing a frequent manifestation of APS in women of childbearing age.

Division of Hematology & Thromboembolism, St Joseph's Hospital, McMaster University, 50 Charlton Avenue, East, Room L208, Hamilton, ON L8N 4A6, Canada
* Corresponding author.
E-mail address: crowthrm@mcmaster.ca

Hematol Oncol Clin N Am 24 (2010) 669–676
doi:10.1016/j.hoc.2010.05.005
0889-8588/10/$ – see front matter
hemonc.theclinics.com

Despite important research efforts over the last 15 years, many questions remain unaddressed, regarding the important aspects of pathophysiology, treatment, and prognosis of this peculiar type of acquired thrombophilia.

EPIDEMIOLOGY

Data on the prevalence of aPL-Abs should be considered with caution, giving the incomplete standardization of methods for their detection. The prevalence of aPL-Abs ranges from 1% to 10% in general population (with an even higher proportion among the elderly) and from about 30% to 40% (and even higher) in patients with SLE.[8] The risk of thrombotic events in asymptomatic patients with aPL-Abs can be up to about 3% per year.[9] Patients presenting with thrombosis have a prevalence of up to 30%.[8] In women with recurrent fetal losses, the proportion of aPL-Abs has been described to vary between 5% and 60%, reflecting again a lack of standardization in aPL-Abs detection (about 15% had persistent aPL-Abs).[10] In unselected women, aPL-Abs were found in 3% to 5%; screening-detected aPL-Abs did not predict poor pregnancy outcome.[10]

PATHOPHYSIOLOGY

aPL-Abs are autoantibodies directed against proteins that bind to anionic phospholipids. Besides APS, aPL-Abs are also found in patients with other conditions including cancer, infections, and in concert with the use of selected medications.[11–14]

Many antigens have been described to be recognized by aPL-Abs, including β_2 glycoprotein I (β_2GPI),[15] prothrombin (PT),[16] protein C complex,[17] annexin A5,[18] proteins of the coagulation cascade (factors VII, XI, XII),[19] and proteins of the fibrinolytic system.[20]

The exact mechanisms by which aPL-Abs cause thrombosis and other clinical manifestations of APS are not understood. The effects of aPL-Abs are directed at different pathways involved in the coagulation process: inhibition of natural anticoagulants and the fibrinolytic system and activation of endothelial cells, platelets, and the complement system.

β_2GPI, a plasma protein with affinity for anionic membrane phospholipids, binds to such membranes with high affinity when aPL-Abs and anti-β_2GPI antibodies are present, affecting the coagulation or fibrinolysis process on those cellular surfaces. Effects may include interference with protein C and other coagulation proteins.[21] Some anticardiolipin antibodies (aCL-Abs) are directed against PT; they may elicit a prothrombotic effect by promoting the activity of PT and interfering with the action of activated protein C (which is a normal indirect inhibitor of thrombin).[17]

aPL-Abs can also react with plasmin, downregulating clot lysis.[22] They may also inhibit the activity of tissue factor pathway inhibitor, an early inhibitor of coagulation activation.[23]

aPL-Abs can also activate endothelial cells, which in turn increase the expression of cellular adhesion molecules and tissue factor, thus enhancing the activation of the coagulation process.[24,25] Finally, the effects of aPL-Abs on platelets include an increase of GpIIb-IIIa expression and increase of thromboxane A_2 synthesis, stimulating platelet aggregation.[11]

The exact mechanism of fetal loss remains still largely unknown. One possible mechanism involves β_2GPI that binds to anionic phospholipids during trophoblast differentiation. When aPL-Abs are present, they can bind to β_2GPI on the membrane of trophoblast cells, thus interfering with adequate placentation.[26] Other possible mechanisms, studied in animal models, involve complement activation (causing fetal damage) and inhibition of annexin A5 (a placental anticoagulant protein) by aPL-Abs.[27]

CLINICAL MANIFESTATIONS

APS has many different clinical manifestations, with a tendency to recur after the initial APS diagnosis. Thrombotic events, involving arteries, veins, or small vessels in any organ or tissue, are the basis of clinical manifestions of APS. In a large, multicenter, international cohort study enrolling 1000 patients with a mean age of 34 years at APS onset, the most frequent thrombotic events at presentation were DVT (31.7%), stroke (13.1%), superficial vein thrombosis (9.1%), PE (9%), TIA (7%), and MI (2.8%).[28]

Other frequent manifestations at onset were thrombocytopenia (21.9%) and livedo reticularis (20.4%); less frequent manifestations were hemolytic anemia, skin ulcers, and pseudovasculitic skin lesions, amaurosis fugax, digital gangrene, and epilepsy. Of note, in this cohort of patients with APS, coexistence of SLE or lupuslike syndrome or other rheumatologic disorders was documented in 47% of patients.[28]

With regard to obstetric manifestations, fetal loss was present in 10% of women as the first clinical manifestation. From APS onset until entry into the study (mean period of evolution, 92 months), 591 women (71.9% of total number of women) experienced at least 1 pregnancy, with 1580 pregnancies in total. Among them, there were 560 (35.4%) early fetal losses (<10 weeks of gestation), 267 (16.9%) late fetal losses (≥10 weeks), and 753 (47.7%) live births (10% of which were premature).[28]

When considering the cumulative clinical features of patients in that cohort, from disease onset until entry into study (mean period of evolution 92 months), venous thromboembolism (VTE), stroke or TIA, MI, fetal losses, livedo reticularis, and thrombocytopenia were still the main clinical manifestations. Of interest, there was a long series of other less-frequent thrombotic events, for example, arterial thrombosis of upper and lower limbs, cerebral venous thrombosis, renal thrombotic manifestations involving renal vein or artery or glomerular vessels, mesenteric ischemia, Budd-Chiari syndrome, and retinal artery and vein thrombosis.

Other less common clinical features deserve some attention, because they were present during the period of evolution in a substantial proportion of patients: migraine (20.2%), epilepsy (7%), cardiac valve thickening or dysfunction (11.6%), amaurosis fugax (5.5%), and hemolytic anemia (9.7%).[28]

APS can also present, at onset or some time after diagnosis, with catastrophic APS (CAPS),[29] which accounts for about 1% of APS cases. Patients with CAPS present with rapidly progressive multiorgan involvement with histopathologic evidence of small vessel occlusions. Despite treatment, CAPS is a life-threatening disease with a mortality of about 50%.[28,30] Data from an ongoing international registry[31] suggest that 46% of patients develop CAPS de novo, without any previous diagnosis of APS. Intra-abdominal manifestations were present in most patients, involving kidney (71%), liver (33%), gastrointestinal tract (25%), spleen (19%), adrenal gland (13%), and pancreas (8%). Pulmonary involvement (mainly acute respiratory distress syndrome and PE) was present in 64% of patients, cerebral manifestations (mainly multiple microinfarctions as well as seizures and headache) in 62%, cardiac disease (cardiac failure, MI, valve lesions) in 51%, and skin complications (livedo reticularis, skin necrosis) in 50%.[31]

DIAGNOSIS

After a preliminary consensus statement was formulated in Sapporo, Japan in 1998,[7] the diagnostic criteria for APS were revised in Sydney, Australia in 2005.[1] The consensus statement contains clinical criteria for thrombotic events and pregnancy complications and laboratory criteria. The diagnosis of APS is confirmed in the presence of at least 1 clinical and 1 laboratory criterion.

Clinical Criteria

1. Vascular thrombosis: one or more venous, arterial, or small vessel thrombotic events in any tissue or organ (superficial vein thrombosis is not included in clinical criteria)
2. Pregnancy morbidity
   One or more unexplained deaths of a morphologically normal fetus at or beyond the 10th week of gestation
   One or more premature births of a morphologically normal neonate before the 34th week of gestation because of eclampsia, severe preeclampsia, or placental insufficiency
   Three or more consecutive spontaneous abortions before the 10th week of gestation (in the absence of parental chromosomal causes and maternal anatomic or hormonal abnormality).

Laboratory Criteria

1. LA present in plasma on 2 or more occasions at least 12 weeks apart (measured according to the guidelines of the International Society on Thrombosis and Haemostasis[32])
2. aCL-Abs (IgG and/or IgM) present in serum or plasma on 2 or more occasions at least 12 weeks apart (in medium or high titer, ie, >40 GPL [IgG phospholipid] or MPL [IgM phospholipid] units or >99th percentile, measured by a standardized enzyme-linked immunosorbent assay [ELISA])
3. Anti-β_2GPI antibody (IgG and/or IgM) present in serum or plasma on 2 or more occasions at least 12 weeks apart (in titer >99th percentile, measured by a standardized ELISA).

The diagnosis of APS cannot be confirmed if less than 12 weeks (or more than 5 years) separate the time of the positive aPL-Ab test and the time of the clinical manifestation.

Moreover, as stated for laboratory criteria, persistence of the aPL-Abs and a second positive test, at least 12 weeks after the first, are required for the diagnosis. To address the issue of epiphenomenal aPL-Abs, the interval required to confirm positivity was increased from 6 weeks (Sapporo criteria) to 12 weeks (revised criteria). However, these intervals are based on expert opinions, confirming the need for validation studies. Coexistence of SLE (or other diseases) distinguishes between primary and secondary APS.

Preliminary diagnostic criteria for CAPS were proposed in 2003:[33]

1. Evidence of involvement of 3 or more organs, systems, and/or tissues
2. Development of manifestations simultaneously or in less than a week
3. Confirmation by histopathology of small vessel occlusion in at least 1 organ or tissue
4. Laboratory confirmation of the presence of aPL-Abs.

The diagnosis of definite CAPS requires all 4 criteria to be fulfilled. In patients without a history of APS, laboratory confirmation of the presence of aPL-Abs must occur and must be confirmed again at least 6 weeks later.

THERAPY

Acute venous or arterial thrombotic events should be treated according to standard recommendations for patients who do not have aPL-Abs. Oral anticoagulant therapy (OAT) effectively prevents recurrent VTE and, perhaps, also arterial thrombosis.[34] Vitamin K antagonists should be administered to achieve an international normalized ratio (INR) between 2 and 3. Higher INR ranges have not proven superior for the prevention of recurrent thrombosis in 2 randomized controlled trials.[35,36]

In a prospective cohort study in patients with a first episode of ischemic stroke and a positive aPL-Ab test, long-term administration of acetylsalicylic acid (ASA; Aspirin) or OAT (administered to an INR of 1.4 to 2.8) was found to be equivalent in the prevention of recurrent stroke.[37] However, it should be noted that aPL-Ab positivity was tested only once in this study and that the risk of recurrent thrombosis was not different between aPL-Abs–positive and aPL-Abs–negative patients (in both warfarin and ASA arms).[37]

The optimal duration of OAT after a first episode of VTE in patients with APS is not known. However, based on observational studies that suggest a high rate of recurrence after warfarin discontinuation, indefinite therapy is suggested.[38]

Whether asymptomatic patients with an aPL-Ab benefit from primary prophylaxis remains a matter of debate. The risk of thrombosis in otherwise healthy persons who were found to be positive for aPL-Abs was very low (<1% per year).[39] A small, randomized controlled trial comparing ASA with placebo in a group of asymptomatic, persistently aPL-Abs–positive individuals did not show any benefit from ASA for the prevention of thrombotic events.[9]

Data are also lacking about thrombotic risk and possible benefits of antithrombotic therapy in nonpregnant women with previous fetal loss and the presence of aPL-Abs but without any previous thrombotic events. In a retrospective study, nonpregnant women diagnosed with APS solely by fetal loss and aPL-Abs positivity, were followed up for 8 years. During follow-up, 10% of women on ASA and 59% of those not on ASA (P<.05) experienced a thrombotic event.[40] The available evidence suggests that either low-dose ASA or no treatment may be used for primary prevention of thrombosis in nonpregnant women diagnosed with APS by pregnancy morbidity and appropriate antibody testing.[34]

The prevention of further pregnancy losses represents the primary therapeutic objective in women with APS diagnosed by aPL-Abs positivity and history of pregnancy loss. Prophylactic dose of heparin (either unfractionated or low molecular weight) in concert with low-dose ASA is currently recommended in clinical practice guidelines.[41]

Treatment of CAPS is not standardized at present, mainly because of the lack of evidence owing to the rarity of this condition. Based on the available evidence, it seems that precipitating factors should be recognized and addressed: infections were found in 22% of patients before CAPS onset.[42] Patients with CAPS should probably receive parenteral anticoagulants when undergoing surgical procedures.[42]

The mainstay of treatment during CAPS is anticoagulant therapy, which should be administered as intravenous heparin. High-dose corticosteroids should be considered in every patient presenting with CAPS. Early addition of plasma exchange and/or intravenous immunoglobulin should be considered in patients who do not respond promptly to heparin and corticosteroids. In the context of an SLE flare, use of cyclophosphamide might also be considered.[31] In the CAPS registry, the highest recovery rate occurred with the combination of anticoagulant, corticosteroids, and plasma exchange.[42]

Finally, rituximab, an anti-CD20 monoclonal antibody, has been used in some case reports and may be useful.[43] Rituximab is currently being studied in a phase II trial, examining anticoagulant-resistant manifestation of APS (http://clinicaltrials.gov/ct2/show/NCT00537290?term=rituximab+antiphospholipid&rank=1).

SUMMARY

APS remains a problematic condition associated with a high risk of morbidity and mortality. Anticoagulant therapy seems to prevent recurrent thrombotic events and may increase the likelihood of successful pregnancy outcomes. At present, there is no evidence to support or refute specific treatment strategies for primary prophylaxis of thrombosis. CAPS is associated with a high risk of mortality and mandates early and aggressive therapy with anticoagulants, immunosuppressive agents, and plasma exchange.

REFERENCES

1. Miyakis S, Lockshin MD, Atsumi T, et al. International Consensus statement on an update of the classification criteria for definite antiphospholipid syndrome (APS). J Thromb Haemost 2006;4:295–306.
2. Soulier MC, Boffa MC. Avortements á répétition, thromboses et anticoagulant circulant antithromboplastine. Nouv Presse Med 1980;9:859–64 [in French].
3. Carreras LO, Defreyn G, Machin SJ, et al. Arterial thrombosis, intrauterine death and "lupus" anticoagulant detection of immunoglobulin interfering with prostacyclin formation. Lancet 1981;1:244–6.
4. Nilsson IM, Astedt B, Hedner U, et al. Intrauterine death and circulating anticoagulant "antithromboplastin". Acta Med Scand 1975;197:153–9.
5. Asherson RA. A 'primary' antiphospholipid syndrome? J Rheumatol 1988;15:1742–6.
6. Font J, Cervera R. Sindrome antifosfolipido primario: una nueva entidad? Med Clin (Barc) 1988;91:736–8 [in Spanish].
7. Wilson WA, Gharavi AE, Koike T, et al. International consensus statement on preliminary classification criteria for definite antiphospholipid syndrome: report of an international workshop. Arthritis Rheum 1999;42:1309–11.
8. Petri M. Epidemiology of the antiphospholipid antibody syndrome. J Autoimmun 2000;15:145–51.
9. Erkan D, Harrison MJ, Levy R, et al. Aspirin for primary thrombosis prevention in the antiphospholipid syndrome: a randomized, double-blind, placebo-controlled trial in asymptomatic antiphospholipid antibody-positive individuals. Arthritis Rheum 2007;56:2382–91.
10. Heilmann L, von Tempelhoff GF, Pollow K. Antiphospholipid syndrome in obstetrics. Clin Appl Thromb Hemost 2003;9:143–50.
11. Palomo I, Segovia F, Ortega C, et al. Antiphospholipid syndrome: a comprehensive review of a complex multisystemic disease. Clin Exp Rheumatol 2009;27:668–77.
12. Levy R, Gharavi A, Sammaritano L, et al. Characteristics of IgG antiphospholipid antibodies in patients with systemic lupus erythematosus and syphilis. J Rheumatol 1990;17:1036–41.
13. Yoon K, Wong A, Shakespeare T, et al. High prevalence of antiphospholipid antibodies in Asian cancer patients with thrombosis. Lupus 2003;12:112–6.
14. Merrill J, Shen C, Gugnani M, et al. High prevalence of antiphospholipid antibodies in patients taking procainamide. J Rheumatol 1997;24:1083–8.

15. Matsuura E, Igarashi Y, Yasuda T, et al. Anticardiolipin antibodies recognize β2-glycoprotein I structure altered by interacting with an oxygen modified solid phase surface. J Exp Med 1994;179:457–62.
16. Bevers E, Galli M, Barbui T, et al. Lupus anticoagulant IgG's (LA) are not directed to phospholipids only, but to a complex of lipid-bound human prothrombin. Thromb Haemost 1991;66:629–32.
17. Galli M, Willems G, Rosing J, et al. Anti-prothrombin IgG from patients with anti-phospholipid antibodies inhibits the inactivation of factor Va by activated protein C. Br J Haematol 2005;129:240–7.
18. Rand J, Wu X. Antibody-mediated interference with annexins in the antiphospholipid syndrome. Thromb Res 2004;114:383–9.
19. Bidot C, Jy W, Horstman L, et al. Factor VII/VIIa: a new antigen in the antiphospholipid antibody syndrome. Br J Haematol 2003;120:618–26.
20. Lopez-Lira F, Rosales-Leon L, Martinez V, et al. The role of β2-glycoprotein I (β2GPI) in the activation of plasminogen. Biochim Biophys Acta 2006;1764:815–23.
21. Safa O, Esmon C, Esmon N. Inhibition of APC anticoagulant activity on oxidized phospholipid by anti-β2-glycoprotein I monoclonal antibodies. Blood 2005;106:1629–35.
22. Yang C, Hwang K, Yan W, et al. Identification of anti-plasmin antibodies in the antiphospholipid syndrome that inhibit degradation of fibrin. J Immunol 2004;172:5765–73.
23. Adams M, Breckler L, Stevens P, et al. Anti-tissue factor pathway inhibitor activity in subjects with antiphospholipid syndrome is associated with increased thrombin generation. Haematologica 2004;89:985–90.
24. Pierangeli S, Espinola R, Liu X, et al. Thrombogenic effects of antiphospholipid antibodies are mediated by intracellular cell adhesion molecue-1, vascular cell adhesion molecule-1, and P-selectin. Circ Res 2001;88:245–50.
25. Pierangeli SS, Harris EN. Probing antiphospholipid-mediated thrombosis: the interplay between anticardiolipin antibodies and endothelial cells. Lupus 2003;12:539–45.
26. Di Simone N, Meroni PL, D'Asta M, et al. Pregnancies complicated with antiphospholipid syndrome: the pathogenic mechanism of antiphospholipid antibodies: a review of the literature. Ann N Y Acad Sci 2007;1108:505–14.
27. Girardi G, Berman J, Redecha P, et al. Complement C5a receptors and neutrophils mediate fetal injury in the antiphospholipid syndrome. J Clin Invest 2003;112:1644–54.
28. Cervera R, Piette JC, Font J, et al. Antiphospholipid syndrome: clinical and immunologic manifestations and patterns of disease expression in a cohort of 1,000 patients. Arthritis Rheum 2002;46:1019–27.
29. Asherson RA. The catastrophic antiphospholipid syndrome. J Rheumatol 1992;19:508–12.
30. Cervera R, Khamashta MA, Shoenfeld Y, et al. Morbidity and mortality in the antiphospholipid syndrome during a 5-year period: a multicentre prospective study of 1000 patients. Ann Rheum Dis 2009;68:1428–32.
31. Cervera R, Bucciarelli S, Plasín MA, et al. Catastrophic antiphospholipid syndrome (CAPS): descriptive analysis of a series of 280 patients from the "CAPS Registry". J Autoimmun 2009;32:240–5.
32. Pengo V, Tripodi A, Reber G, et al. Update of the guidelines for lupus anticoagulant detection. J Thromb Haemost 2009;7:1737–40.
33. Asherson RA, Cervera R, de Groot PG, et al. Catastrophic antiphospholipid syndrome: international consensus statement on classification criteria and treatment guidelines. Lupus 2003;12:530–4.

34. Lim W, Crowther MA, Eikelboom JW. Management of antiphospholipid antibody syndrome: a systematic review. JAMA 2006;295:1050–7.
35. Crowther MA, Ginsberg JS, Julian J, et al. A comparison of two intensities of warfarin for the prevention of recurrent thrombosis in patients with the antiphospholipid antibody syndrome. N Engl J Med 2003;349:1133–8.
36. Finazzi G, Marchioli R, Brancaccio V, et al. A randomized clinical trial of high-intensity warfarin vs conventional antithrombotic therapy for the prevention of recurrent thrombosis in patients with the antiphospholipid syndrome (WASP). J Thromb Haemost 2005;3:848–53.
37. Levine SR, Brey RL, Tilley BC, et al. Antiphospholipid antibodies and subsequent thrombo-occlusive events in patients with ischemic stroke. JAMA 2004;291: 576–84.
38. Ruiz-Irastorza G, Hunt BJ, Khamashta MA. A systematic review of secondary thromboprophylaxis in patients with antiphospholipid antibodies. Arthritis Rheum 2007;57:1487–95.
39. Vila P, Hernandez MC, Lopez-Fernandez MF, et al. Prevalence, follow-up and clinical significance of the anticardiolipin antibodies in normal subjects. Thromb Haemost 1994;72:209–13.
40. Erkan D, Merrill JT, Yazici Y, et al. High thrombosis rate after fetal loss in antiphospholipid syndrome: effective prophylaxis with aspirin. Arthritis Rheum 2001;44: 1466–7.
41. Bates SM, Greer IA, Pabinger I, et al. Venous thromboembolism, thrombophilia, antithrombotic therapy, and pregnancy: American College of Chest Physicians Evidence-Based Clinical Practice Guidelines (8th edition). Chest 2008;133: 844S–86S.
42. Bucciarelli S, Espinosa G, Cervera R. The CAPS registry: morbidity and mortality of the catastrophic antiphospholipid syndrome. Lupus 2009;18:905–12.
43. Ramos-Casals M, Brito-Zerón P, Muñoz S, et al. A systematic review of the off-label use of biological therapies in systemic autoimmune diseases. Medicine (Baltimore) 2008;87:345–64.

Pulmonary Embolism in Medical-Surgical Critically Ill Patients

Deborah J. Cook, MD[a,b,*], Marco P. Donadini, MD[a,c]

KEYWORDS

- Pulmonary embolism • Thromboprophylaxis
- Critically ill patients • Medical-surgical ICU

VENOUS THROMBOEMBOLISM DURING CRITICAL ILLNESS

Venous thromboembolism (VTE), which includes deep vein thrombosis (DVT) and pulmonary embolism (PE), is a common complication of critical illness.[1,2] Most thrombi are asymptomatic and are confined to the deep veins of the calf. However, with time, 20% to 30% of untreated calf vein thrombi extend proximally into the thigh, where, if untreated, they pose a 40% to 50% risk of PE.[3] Early studies of the natural history of PE suggest that untreated PE has a 25% mortality rate.[4]

Although DVT has potentially serious consequences, it is often unrecognized in critically ill patients. In an observational study of 100 patients admitted to the intensive care unit (ICU), lower limb Doppler ultrasonography was performed twice weekly.[5] In these patients, whose type of thromboprophylaxis was selected by physicians, DVT was diagnosed in 32% of those receiving no intervention, in 40% of those receiving subcutaneous unfractionated heparin (UFH), and in 33% of those receiving mechanical prophylaxis (antiembolic stockings or pneumatic compression devices). Concern about undiagnosed VTE in the medical-surgical ICU setting is underscored by studies showing that 10%[6] to 100%[5,7] of DVTs found by ultrasonographic screening were not detected on physical examination. In a study of lower limb ultrasonographic screening done twice weekly in medical-surgical ICU patients, proximal DVT occurred in 25 of 261 (9.6%) patients during the ICU stay and in 4 additional patients after ICU discharge, accounting for a total of 29 of 261 (11.1%) patients. All

Dr Cook holds a Research Chair of the Canadian Institutes for Health Research, Ottawa, Ontario, Canada.

[a] Department of Medicine, McMaster University, Hamilton, ON L8N3Z5, Canada
[b] Department of Clinical Epidemiology and Biostatistics, McMaster University, Hamilton, ON L8N3Z5, Canada
[c] Division of Hematology & Thromboembolism, St Joseph's Hospital, McMaster University, 50 Charlton Avenue, East, Room L208, Hamilton, ON L8N 4A6, Canada
* Corresponding author. Department of Medicine, McMaster University, Hamilton, ON L8N3Z5, Canada.
E-mail address: debcook@mcmaster.ca

Hematol Oncol Clin N Am 24 (2010) 677–682
doi:10.1016/j.hoc.2010.05.002
0889-8588/10/$ – see front matter © 2010 Published by Elsevier Inc.

but one case of DVT was clinically unsuspected, and all cases occurred despite routine heparin thromboprophylaxis.[8]

Clinically unsuspected PE may also have catastrophic consequences in ICU patients. Mechanically ventilated patients who have sudden hypoxemia, hypotension, or tachycardia may have undetected PE.[9] PE may also contribute to difficulty in weaning patients from mechanical ventilation.[5] In ICU patients with impaired cardiopulmonary reserve, even a small PE might have severe or fatal consequences.[10] In one study, 13 of 34 (38.2%) critically ill patients with known DVT and no symptoms of PE had PE diagnosed by ventilation-perfusion scans.[11] In an autopsy study, PE was found in 59 of 404 (15%) hospitalized patients. In another autopsy study, PE was unsuspected during antemortem in 14 of 20 (70%) patients who died of PE.[12] In a 25-year longitudinal study, 9% of patients had PE at autopsy, but in 84% of these patients, the antemortem diagnosis was missed.[13]

In summary, DVT and PE are common in ICU patients; PE remains one of the most common unsuspected autopsy findings in critically ill patients.[14]

THROMBOPROPHYLAXIS IN MEDICAL-SURGICAL ICU PATIENTS

Given the high prevalence of VTE and the potential morbidity and mortality associated with PE, it follows that if VTE prophylaxis is effective, it should be used in the ICU.[2] The beneficial effect of subcutaneous UFH to prevent VTE has long been established.[15] In 2 meta-analyses of trials enrolling more than 8000 patients who underwent general surgery, UFH resulted in a 60% to 70% relative risk reduction for DVT and fatal PE.[16,17] Strategies to prevent VTE are of proven benefit in multiple patient populations, are widely available, and have a low risk of toxicity.

However, only 2 randomized clinical trials have compared active thromboprophylaxis with placebo in critically ill medical-surgical patients.[18,19] One double-blind randomized trial allocated 199 medical-surgical ICU patients to a twice-daily subcutaneous administration of UFH, 5000 IU, or placebo.[18] Using serial fibrinogen leg scanning for 5 days, the DVT rates were found to be 13% in the UFH group and 29% in the placebo group (relative risk reduction being 0.65). Rates of bleeding, PE, and mortality were not reported. Subsequent demonstration that leg scanning is not a reliable diagnostic test for DVT limits the utility of this study.[20,21] In a multicenter trial, Fraisse and colleagues[19] randomized 223 patients mechanically ventilated for chronic obstructive pulmonary disease to a once-daily administration of the low-molecular-weight heparin (LMWH), nadroparin, or placebo. Patients had weekly ultrasonography, and venography was recommended at 21 days or earlier if results from ultrasonography were positive or nondiagnostic. The proportion of patients developing DVT was 16% in the nadroparin group and 28% in the placebo group (relative risk reduction being 0.45). There was a trend toward increased overall bleeding (25 vs 18 patients, $P = .18$) and major hemorrhage (6 vs 3 patients, $P = .28$) in the nadroparin group. PE was not systematically evaluated; 8 patients in each group died ($P = .72$), but autopsies were not performed.

In summary, the beneficial effect of thromboprophylaxis on DVT in medical-surgical patients has been documented. However, whether thromboprophylaxis decreases PE rates alone has not been directly determined in randomized trials because of the small sample sizes of the available trials and because only few patients were diagnosed with PE.

DIAGNOSING PE

The reference standard for the diagnosis of PE is contrast pulmonary angiography. However, contrast pulmonary angiography is rarely performed in the ICU because of technical difficulty, cost, potential for toxicity, and the difficulty of transporting critically ill patients to the radiology department. Computed tomographic pulmonary angiography (CTPA) has replaced direct pulmonary angiography because of its ease of use and widespread availability; however, CTPA is expensive and is associated with the same transport risk and risk of contrast-induced nephropathy. CTPA has a sensitivity of 83% and a specificity of 95%[22] in hospitalized patients. Ventilation-perfusion lung scanning, although widely used outside the ICU, is not too useful during critical illness, because ventilation cannot be easily performed in mechanically ventilated patients, and a prevalent pulmonary pathologic condition in the ICU often creates indeterminate results. Other tests such as transthoracic echocardiography showing features such as dilatation of the right side of the heart are suggestive but not diagnostic of PE.

Because pulmonary angiography and CTPA are performed in only a small proportion of critically ill patients who are deemed stable for transport and unlikely to develop contrast nephropathy and because lung scans are rarely interpretable, a large proportion of critically ill patients who have clinical signs of PE do not undergo objective testing. Such patients are either treated empirically or diagnosis is considered but not pursued because of the lack of a safe, available, and validated evaluative regimen; that is, in addition to the low pretest probability of PE in the ICU setting, there is a low rate of objective testing in practice.

As demonstrated in trauma patients, the diagnosis of PE is very challenging during critical illness. In a trauma ICU, 48 of 972 patients with a 10% or greater sudden decrease in oxygen saturation (Sao_2) but no changes in static lung compliance underwent pulmonary arteriography (PA)[23]; 21of 48 (44%) had PE on a PA test and either a clear chest radiograph or no change in previous pulmonary pathology. Investigators suggested that trauma patients who have more than 10% decrease in Sao_2 without changes in lung compliance or chest radiograph findings should undergo PA—an approach, which yields a sensitivity, specificity, and predictive value of 100%, 99.9%, and 95%, respectively, for the diagnosis of clinically significant PE. However, performing PA in all medical-surgical critically ill patients who have greater than 10% decrease in Sao_2 and no change in lung compliance or chest radiograph findings is premature for the medical-surgical ICU population.

In clinical trials, because of the difficulty in interpreting some test results, central adjudication is often used to categorize PE outcomes. For blinded and unblinded trials in which outcome ascertainment bias is minimal, and when objective outcomes are measured, adjudication is generally unnecessary. However, outcome adjudication for events such as PE is desirable because the outcome is subject to ascertainment bias; clinical definitions vary, creating poor reproducibility; and outcome assessment requires specialized knowledge, making misclassification common. In such circumstances, PE is sometimes classified as follows: (1) definite PE, (2) probable PE, (3) possible PE, and (4) no PE. Common definitions are definite PE: clearly positive test result without reference to a clinical suspicion or pretest probability, probable PE: moderate to high pretest probability (high clinical suspicion) plus no test or a nondiagnostic test, possible PE: low pretest probability (low clinical suspicion) plus a nondiagnostic test, and no PE: clearly negative test result.

In summary, PE is underdiagnosed during critical illness because of the nonspecific nature of the presentation, low rates of testing, and challenging test-result interpretation. For clinical trial purposes, patients with suspected PE often undergo adjudication by a blinded review committee. Typically, PE is diagnosed by an intraluminal filling defect on either chest computed tomography (CT) or direct pulmonary angiogram. For those critically ill patients who are not mechanically ventilated, segmental or greater perfusion defects on lung scans, with a normal chest radiograph in the area of the defect are also diagnosed as having PE in the setting of a compatible clinical history.

RISK FACTORS AND CONSEQUENCES OF DVT AND PE IN THE ICU

In a screening study for DVT in medical-surgical ICU patients, the authors found 4 independent DVT risk factors, including 2 baseline characteristics: (1) personal or family history of DVT (hazard ratio [HR] 4.0; 95% confidence interval [CI], 1.5–10.3) and (2) end-stage, dialysis-dependent renal failure (HR 3.7; 95% CI, 1.2–11.1) and 2 ICU-acquired exposures: platelet transfusion (HR 3.2; 95% CI, 1.2–8.4) and vaso-pressor use (HR 2.8; 95% CI, 1.1–7.2). When compared with patients without DVT, patients with DVT had longer durations of mechanical ventilation (median of 9 vs 6 days, P = .03), ICU stay (median 17.5 vs 9 days, P = .005), and hospital stay (median of 51 vs 23 days, P<.001).[8] Mortality in ICU (25.0% vs 27.3%) and hospital (53.1% vs 37.4%) were not statistically different.

A prospective single-center study of patients with severe congestive heart failure (CHF) admitted to a coronary care unit, determined the incidence of and risk factors for clinical PE using high-probability lung scans, chest CT, or pulmonary angiography.[24] Of the 198 patients recruited, 18 patients (9.1%) had PE in hospital, and DVT was demonstrated in 8 of these 18 patients (44.4%) with PE. Patients with and without PE were similar with respect to age, sex, CHF severity, and comorbidities. In logistic regression, only cancer (odds ratio [OR] 26.9; 95% CI, 4.9–146.8), right ventricle abnormality (OR 9.7; 95% CI, 2.2–42.6), and previous VTE (OR 9.1; 95% CI, 1.28–64.7) were independently associated with PE.

In summary, in contrast to DVT, there are no ICU-specific data for patients with and without PE to calculate estimated baseline and time-dependent independent risk factors for PE and the attributable morbidity and mortality of PE.

PE TREATMENT

Patients with echocardiographic findings that are consistent with massive PE and patients with significant cardiovascular compromise usually receive either direct or systemic thrombolysis. However, most critically ill patients are treated with intravenous UFH, and a small proportion of them are treated with a subcutaneous therapeutic dose of LMWH. Patients perceived to have a high risk of bleeding may be monitored for cardiopulmonary deterioration or treated with insertion of an inferior vena caval filter. Without treatment, patients may develop progressive thromboses or die. Some patients may survive despite no treatment, depending on their clot burden and cardiopulmonary reserve.

In summary, the management of all VTE events is at the discretion of the ICU team, and therapies are variable. To the authors' knowledge there are no studies documenting PE treatments or the determinants of PE treatment in the ICU setting.

PE OUTCOME PREDICTION

Reliable prediction of adverse outcomes in acute PE may help choose between in-hospital and ambulatory treatment for patients presenting to the emergency department. Wicki and colleagues[25] aimed to identify predictors of adverse events in patients with PE and to generate a simple risk score. The investigators prospectively followed up 296 patients with PE admitted to the emergency department. Logistic regression was used to predict death, recurrent VTE, or major bleeding at 3 months. Factors associated with an adverse outcome in multivariate analysis were cancer, heart failure, previous DVT, systolic blood pressure less than 100 mm Hg, and Pao_2 less than 8 kPa. A risk score was calculated by adding 2 points each for cancer and hypotension and 1 point each for the other predictors. Investigators concluded that a simple score might accurately identify patients with PE in the emergency department who are at low risk of an adverse outcome. Such a score may be useful for selecting patients with PE who can be triaged for outpatient care. However, this score was neither developed nor tested in hospitalized patients and may not be applicable to ICU patients.

In another study of patients admitted to hospital, the investigators randomly allocated 15,531 inpatient discharges with PE from 186 hospitals to either derivation (67%) or internal validation (33%) samples, to develop a clinical prediction rule that accurately classifies patients with PE into categories of increasing risk of mortality and other adverse medical outcomes.[26] The prediction rule was derived using logistic regression with 30-day mortality as the primary outcome, using 11 demographic and clinical variables that are routinely available as potential predictor variables. The rule was externally validated in 221 inpatients with PE. The prediction rule accurately classifies patients with PE into 5 groups of increasing risk of mortality and other adverse medical outcomes; however, further validation is needed. This rule is not likely directly applicable to critically ill patients already receiving advanced life support in the ICU.

In summary, there are no PE outcome prediction models that have been developed for the ICU setting or adapted to medical-surgical ICU patients. However, a simple, objective set of factors that predict outcome for critically ill patients with PE could provide helpful information to guide prognosis discussions by clinicians with families. Such factors could guide the venue of care (intermediate step-down unit or ICU) and initial treatment.

FUTURE RESEARCH

More investigations are needed on PE in medical-surgical ICU patients, including issues on the epidemiologic aspects of PE (including risk factors and attributable morbidity and mortality) and treatment of PE (including pharmacologic and nonpharmacologic approaches, determinants of treatment variation, and predictors of PE outcome adjusted for treatment). Therefore, a research agenda is required to focus on PE in medical-surgical ICU patients to address some of these knowledge gaps.

REFERENCES

1. Attia J, Ray JG, Cook DJ, et al. Deep vein thrombosis and its prevention in critically ill patients. Arch Intern Med 2001;161(10):1268–79.
2. Geerts WH, Bergqvist D, Pineo GF, et al. Prevention of venous thromboembolism: American College of Chest Physicians Evidence-Based Clinical Practice Guidelines. (8th edition). Chest 2008;133(Suppl 6):381S–453S.
3. Kakkar VV, Flanc C, Howe CT, et al. Natural history of postoperative deep vein thrombosis. Lancet 1969;2:230–2.
4. Barritt DW, Jordan SC. Anticoagulant drugs in the treatment of pulmonary embolism: a controlled trial. Lancet 1960;i:1309–12.
5. Hirsh DR, Ingenito EP, Goldhaber SZ. Prevalence of deep venous thrombosis among patients in medical intensive care. JAMA 1995;274:335–7.
6. Marik PE, Andrews L, Maini B. The incidence of deep venous thrombosis in ICU patients. Chest 1997;111:661–4.
7. Harris LM, Curl RC, Booth FV, et al. Screening for asymptomatic deep vein thrombosis in surgical intensive care patients. J Vasc Surg 1997;26:764–9.

8. Cook DJ, Crowther M, Meade M, et al. Deep venous thrombosis in medical-surgical critically ill patients: prevalence, incidence and risk factors. Crit Care Med 2005;33(7):1565–71.

9. McKelvie PA. Autopsy evidence of pulmonary thromboembolism. Med J Aust 1994;160:127–8.

10. Douketis JD, Foster GA, Crowther MA, et al. Clinical risk factors and timing of recurrent venous thromboembolism during the initial 3 months of anticoagulant therapy. Arch Intern Med 2000;160(22):3431–6.

11. Moser KM, LeMoine JR, Nachtwey FJ, et al. Deep venous thrombosis and pulmonary embolism: frequency in a respiratory intensive care unit. JAMA 1981;246:1422–4.

12. Stein PD, Henry JW. Prevalence of acute pulmonary embolism among patients in a general hospital and at autopsy. Chest 1995;108:978–81.

13. Karwinski B, Svendsen E. Comparison of clinical and postmortem diagnosis of pulmonary embolism. J Clin Pathol 1989;42:135–9.

14. Twigg SJ, McCrirrick A, Sanderson PM. A comparison of post mortem findings with post hoc estimated clinical diagnoses of patients who die in a United Kingdom intensive care unit. Intensive Care Med 2001;27:706–10.

15. Halkin H, Goldberg J, Modan M, et al. Reduction of mortality in general medical in-patients by low-dose heparin prophylaxis. Ann Intern Med 1982;96:561–5.

16. Clagett GP, Reisch JS. Prevention of venous thromboembolism in general surgical patients. Ann Surg 1988;208(2):227–40.

17. Collins R, Scrimgeour A, Yusuf S, et al. Reduction in fatal pulmonary embolism and venous thrombosis by perioperative administration of subcutaneous heparin. N Engl J Med 1988;318(18):1162–73.

18. Cade JF. High risk of the critically ill for venous thromboembolism. Crit Care Med 1982;10:448–50.

19. Fraisse F, Holzapfel L, Couland JM, et al. Nadroparin in the prevention of deep vein thrombosis in acute decompensated COPD. The Association of Non-University Affiliated Intensive Care Specialist Physicians in France. Am J Respir Crit Care Med 2000;161:1109–14.

20. Cruickshank MK, Levine MN, Hirsh J, et al. An evaluation of impedance plethysmography and ^{125}I-fibrinogen leg scanning in patients following hip surgery. Thromb Haemost 1989;62:830–4.

21. Lensing AW, Hirsh J. ^{125}I-fibrinogen leg scanning: reassessment of its role for the diagnosis of venous thrombosis in post-operative patients. Thromb Haemost 1993;69:2–7.

22. Stein PD, Fowler SE, Goodman LR, et al, PIOPED II Investigators. Multidetector computed tomography for acute pulmonary embolism. N Engl J Med 2006;354(22):2317–27.

23. Brathwaite CEM, O'Malley KF, Ross SE, et al. Continuous pulse oximetry and the diagnosis of pulmonary embolism in critically ill trauma patients. J Trauma 1992;33(4):528–31.

24. Darze ES, Latado AL, Guimara AG, et al. Incidence and clinical predictors of pulmonary embolism in severe heart failure patients admitted to a coronary care unit. Chest 2005;128:2576–80.

25. Wicki J, Perrier A, Perneger TV, et al. Predicting adverse outcome in patients with acute pulmonary embolism: a risk score. Thromb Haemost 2000;84:548–52.

26. Aujesky D, Obrosky DS, Stone RA, et al. Derivation and validation of a prognostic model for pulmonary embolism. Am J Respir Crit Care Med 2005;172:1041–6.

Prevention and Treatment of Hormone-Associated Venous Thromboembolism: A Patient Management Approach

Joanna Ueng, MD, James D. Douketis, MD, FRCP(C)*

KEYWORDS

- Venous thromboembolism • Hormonal therapy
- Oral contraceptives • Hormone replacement therapy

Hormonal therapy is a common therapeutic agent used by women in the form of the oral contraceptive (OC) or hormone replacement therapy (HRT). An estimated 100 million women use a typical OC consisting of an estrogen and a progestin component, which is also available as transdermal and vaginal ring formulations.[1] Approximately 13 million women use a progestin-only contraceptive, which has comparable contraceptive efficacy as the combined estrogen-progestin formulations and is available in oral, intramuscular, intrauterine, and subdermal formulations.[2] HRT, which can be defined as an estrogen with or without a progestin that is given in oral or transdermal forms, is an effective treatment for menopausal symptoms such as vasomotor flushing and mood instability, and is recommended for short-term (<2 year) use in such patients.[3,4] Transdermal HRT is widely used in Europe, whereas its use in North America is infrequent.[5] In addition to systemic HRT, topical hormone replacement is available as an estrogen cream, an estradiol-containing vaginal ring and an estradiol-containing vaginal tablet and is an effective treatment for menopause-related vaginal symptoms such as vulvar and vaginal atrophy.[4,5]

In the past decade, observational studies[6–12] and randomized controlled trials[13,14] have established that HRT is associated with a two- to threefold increased risk of developing venous thromboembolism (VTE), which includes deep vein thrombosis and pulmonary embolism. A few clinical studies have compared the risk for VTE between oral and transdermal HRT,[4,8,9] with an approximately twofold higher risk

Department of Medicine, St Joseph's Healthcare Hamilton, McMaster University, Room F-544, 50 Charlton Avenue East, Hamilton, ON L8N 4A6, Canada
* Corresponding author.
E-mail address: jdouket@mcmaster.ca

Hematol Oncol Clin N Am 24 (2010) 683–694
doi:10.1016/j.hoc.2010.05.008
0889-8588/10/$ – see front matter © 2010 Elsevier Inc. All rights reserved.

for VTE with transdermal HRT reported in 2 case-control studies.[8,9] However, these studies were small, and a five- to sevenfold increased risk for VTE with transdermal HRT could not be excluded. In another, larger, case-control study, there was an increased risk for VTE in users of oral HRT (hazard ratio [HR] = 3.5; 95% confidence interval [CI]: 1.8–6.8), but no increased risk for VTE in users of transdermal HRT (HR = 0.9; 95% CI: 0.5–1.6).[15] A possible explanation for the clinical and biochemical differences between oral and transdermal HRT may be that transdermal HRT bypasses first-pass hepatic metabolism that occurs with oral HRT.[16,17]

In women who use OCs, the risk of VTE is approximately two- to fourfold higher than that among those who do not use OCs, as demonstrated in 43 case-control studies since 1967,[10,18–58] 3 prospective cohort studies,[59–61] and 1 randomized controlled trial.[62] However, the estimated absolute risk of developing VTE remains low, increasing from 1 per 10,000 person-years, to 2 to 4 per 10,000 person-years during the time when the OC is used. Interestingly, several studies have shown that the absolute risk for VTE in women who use OCs and have a prothrombotic blood disorder, such as the factor V Leiden or prothrombin gene G20210A mutations, is higher than expected from the addition of these risks, thereby suggesting a possible enhancement in their individual effect on thrombosis risk.[63–67]

Little is known about the risk of VTE associated with the use of topical (vaginal) hormone replacement, as there are no published studies that specifically address this question. Systemic absorption is minimal with topical estrogen,[68–73] suggesting that the risk of VTE may not be increased among users of topical estrogen therapy compared with nonusers. In addition, studies of OC use show that the risk of VTE is approximately twice as high in users of OCs containing higher estrogen doses in comparison with users of OCs containing lower estrogen doses;[26,31] thus, the very low doses of estrogen commonly used for the effective treatment of the vaginal symptoms of menopause (ie, 0.3 mg conjugated equine estrogen per day for estrogen cream, 5–10 μg estrogen released per day for estradiol-containing vaginal ring and 25 μg estrogen per day for estradiol-containing vaginal tablet)[5] may not be associated with an increased risk of VTE. However, more research is needed before firm conclusions can be made regarding the safety of topical (vaginal) hormone replacement.

Given the known increased risk of VTE associated with both OC use and HRT use, it is important to address questions about the prevention and management of hormone-associated VTE. Specifically, the objectives of this article are as follows: (1) to provide suggested clinical management approaches for the primary and secondary prevention of VTE for women with thrombophilia; (2) to provide suggested clinical management approaches for the primary and secondary prevention of VTE in the perioperative period for women taking the OC or HRT; and (3) to provide practical management approaches for frequently encountered clinical scenarios relating to duration of treatment for hormone-associated VTE.

IS SCREENING FOR THROMBOPHILIA INDICATED FOR WOMEN WHO WILL BE STARTING HORMONE THERAPY?

In women with thrombophilia, use of either OCs or HRT is associated with an increased risk of VTE.[63–67,74,75] Given this increased risk, it may be a reasonable strategy to screen for thrombophilia before starting hormone therapy. However, a universal screening program for thrombophilia in women who are planning to take or who are already receiving an OC may not be feasible to prevent fatal VTE.[63] For example, Vandenbroucke and associates[63] have inferred that 400,000 women would have to be screened for the factor V Leiden mutation to prevent one VTE-related death. These investigators used an estimated annual incidence of VTE among factor V Leiden carriers who use the OC of 28.5 per 10,000 woman years and assumed a case-fatality rate of 2%, thereby estimating an annual death rate of 5.7 per 100,000. Thus, universal genetic screening before starting hormone therapy does not appear to be justified. Instead, a more reasonable approach would involve selective screening in women for whom there is an increased clinical index of suspicion for thrombophilia, such as a personal history of VTE or family history of VTE in first-degree relatives, consisting of parents and siblings.

SHOULD HORMONE THERAPY BE STARTED IN WOMEN WITH THROMBOPHILIA?
Women Considering an OC

In women with asymptomatic thrombophilia who do not have a prior history of VTE, counseling should be provided on the risk of OC-associated VTE and on alternative forms of contraception with the aim that the patient will partake in the clinical decision-making process. This open discussion is warranted because the risk of OC-associated VTE will vary depending on the prothrombotic blood abnormality. Thus, in heterozygous carriers of the factor V Leiden or prothrombin G20210A mutations, the risk for VTE, although greatly increased relative to nonusers of the OC, should be weighed against potential health benefits of the OC. This can be better achieved if the absolute risk of VTE with OC use is considered in such patients, which is 28 to 50 cases per 10,000 woman-years of OC use.[63] This risk may be considered acceptable for some women and unacceptably high for others. The risk should be weighed against the health and social consequences of unplanned pregnancy if the OC is not used. In healthy women, VTE is more frequent during pregnancy than during OC use, with an estimated incidence of 1 case per 1000 deliveries and a 1% to 2% case-fatality rate.[64,65]

In women with a deficiency of antithrombin III or protein C, it is prudent to avoid OCs because of the reported absolute risk for VTE with OC use of 400 per 10,000 patient-years of OC use.[66] The OC-related VTE risk in carriers of protein S deficiency is uncertain but is likely comparably increased to that with other deficiencies of endogenous anticoagulants.

Another management option for contraception in women with asymptomatic thrombophilia is a progestin-only contraceptive. These preparations may be associated with a lower risk for VTE compared with combined estrogen-progestin OCs, presumably because the estrogen component of the OC is considered to harbor the prothrombotic effects.[67] However, there are no studies that have addressed the safety of progestin-only contraceptives in women with asymptomatic thrombophilia or a history of VTE.

In women with symptomatic thrombophilia, that is, with prior VTE that occurred in association with a prothrombotic blood abnormality, OC use should generally be avoided. If an OC is used, consideration should be given for patients to receive coadministered antithrombotic therapy. One option is to use warfarin, administered to achieve an international normalized ratio (INR) range of 2.0 to 3.0, in combination with the OC. The antithrombotic effects of warfarin are likely to neutralize any prothrombotic effects of the OC given that, in relative terms, OC therapy is a weak risk factor for VTE. However, this approach, although reasonable, has not been assessed in prospective clinical trials. An alternative management approach may be use of low-dose low-molecular-weight heparin (LMWH) therapy in combination with the OC, which has advantages over warfarin therapy of not requiring laboratory monitoring, but has disadvantages relating to greater costs and the potential for heparin-induced osteopenia with long-term use.[76] As with combined OC-warfarin therapy, the efficacy and safety of this management strategy have not been evaluated in prospective clinical trials.

Women Considering HRT

In otherwise healthy patients who are asymptomatic carriers of the factor V Leiden mutation, the risk of a first episode of VTE is four- to fivefold higher than the risk in patients without this mutation. In women who are asymptomatic carriers of the factor V Leiden mutation and are receiving HRT, the risk for a first episode of VTE is 7- to 17-fold higher than in patients without the factor V Leiden mutation who are not receiving HRT.[77,78,79] Based on these relative risk estimates, the absolute risk for VTE can be determined based on individual patient characteristics. For example, in a patient who is a heterozygous carrier of the factor V Leiden mutation who is commencing treatment with HRT, the annual risk for VTE is estimated at 0.7% to 1.5% per year. Thus, for every 65 to 130 patients treated with HRT, 1 patient will develop VTE per year.

Estimating the risk of VTE with HRT use in women with other prothrombotic blood abnormalities is problematic because of a lack of relevant data. Compared with carriers of the factor V Leiden mutation, the risk for VTE appears less in carriers of the prothrombin mutation, and one can estimate the annual risk for VTE at less than 0.7% per year.[80] In patients with deficiencies of the endogenous anticoagulants, protein C, protein S, and antithrombin, there are no data to provide estimates of risk for VTE. However, such patients have a high lifetime risk of developing VTE, which is up to 50% by the fourth or fifth decade of life.[80] Consequently, it is likely that exposure to HRT in such patients will be associated with a high absolute risk for VTE, irrespective of the additive effect of HRT on this risk. In patients with elevated factor VIII, factor IX, factor XI, or hyperhomocysteinemia, data are lacking to make inferences about risk for VTE, either in nonusers or users of HRT. Finally, in patients with antiphospholipid antibodies, which includes the lupus anticoagulant or anticardiolipin antibodies, there is also a lack of data to make inferences about VTE risk. However, such patients also may be at high risk for a first episode of VTE, particularly in patients with systemic lupus erythematosus, and can be considered similar to patients with deficiencies of endogenous anticoagulants.

Thus, the risk of a first VTE when starting HRT is likely to be high in patients with a deficiency of endogenous anticoagulants; moderate to high in patients with factor V Leiden or prothrombin mutations; and uncertain in patients with elevated factor VIII, factor IX, factor XI, or hyperhomocysteinemia.

The approach to women with symptomatic thrombophilia who are interested in HRT is similar to that taken for women considering an OC. Namely, HRT should generally be avoided in women with prior VTE. This includes women who are interested in transdermal HRT. Although transdermal HRT may be associated with a lower or, possibly, no increased risk for VTE compared with oral HRT, extrapolating this premise to women with previous VTE should be done with caution. In any case, if HRT is used, coadministered antithrombotic therapy with warfarin or LMWH may be used. As with coadministered antithrombotic and OC therapy, the safety and efficacy of this management strategy has not been formally evaluated with prospective clinical trials.

WHAT IS THE PERIOPERATIVE MANAGEMENT OF WOMEN WHO ARE USING HORMONAL THERAPY AND WHO ARE UNDERGOING ELECTIVE SURGERY?

To date, there is no compelling evidence from studies of users of the OC or HRT who require elective surgery that hormonal therapy needs to be temporarily discontinued before and after surgery. Some experts suggest that there is the potential that perioperative use of an OC will further increase the risk for lower limb deep vein thrombosis (DVT) beyond that conferred by the surgical procedure and postoperative immobility.[61,67] A prospective cohort study found a nonstatistically significant doubling of the risk of postoperative DVT in women who used an OC during the month of surgery compared with those who stopped their OC use more than 1 month before surgery.[61] However, the absolute incidence of postoperative DVT in young women remains low and the OC is a relatively weak risk factor for DVT compared with the risk associated with surgery alone and any possible additive effect of the OC is unlikely to be important in terms of the overall DVT risk.

Among users of HRT, a similar uncertainty exists as to whether HRT should be temporarily interrupted in the perioperative period.[81,82] Although there is the potential that perioperative use of HRT will further increase the risk for DVT beyond that conferred by the surgical procedure and postoperative immobility, HRT is a relatively weak risk factor for DVT compared with the risk associated with surgery. Thus, any possible additive effect of HRT may not be important in terms of the overall risk. In fact, it has been shown that there is a two- to threefold increased in risk for DVT in users of HRT compared with nonusers, whereas there is a 40- to 50-fold increased risk for DVT in patients undergoing elective major orthopedic surgery compared with those not undergoing surgery.[83] Recent studies further suggest that perioperative use of HRT is not associated with a significant increase in the risk for postoperative VTE. In a case-control study of 318 postmenopausal women (108 cases, 210 controls) who underwent hip or knee replacement surgery, there was no significant difference in the incidence of postoperative VTE in women who received perioperative HRT and women who did not receive perioperative HRT (17% vs 23%; odds ratio [OR] = 0.66; 95% CI: 0.35–1.18).[84] In another case-control study that assessed 1168 women with DVT (256 cases, 912 controls), a subgroup of which had DVT occurring after exposure to a transient risk factor such as surgery or immobility, HRT use was not associated with an increased risk for DVT (OR = 1.17; 95% CI: 0.51–2.72).[85]

Overall, in users of hormone therapy who require elective surgery, there is no compelling evidence that the hormone therapy needs to be discontinued in the perioperative period; however, appropriate methods of thromboprophylaxis should be considered in patients with other strong risk factors for VTE, such as prior VTE, or anticipated prolonged postoperative immobility. In these patients, appropriate management may include temporarily discontinuing the OC or HRT before and after surgery.

WHAT IS THE MANAGEMENT OF PATIENTS WITH HORMONE-ASSOCIATED VTE?
Initial Management

Women who develop VTE while using an OC should discontinue the OC, at least temporarily for 3 months or longer. Indirect evidence suggests that VTE which occurs during the use of an OC is less likely to recur when OCs are stopped, because stopping the OC may have the effect of removing an ongoing prothrombotic stimulus.[34,35] Anticoagulant therapy should be started as in women who develop VTE without associated OC use. Oral anticoagulants, administered to achieve an INR of 2.0 to 3.0, should be initiated together with a therapeutic-dose of unfractionated heparin or LMWH. Heparin can be discontinued after at least 4 to 6 days of therapy and when the INR is higher than 2.0 for two consecutive days.

For women who develop VTE while using HRT, it is generally accepted that HRT should be stopped as there are few clinical situations that would warrant ongoing HRT in the face of newly diagnosed VTE. One such situation might be patients who have debilitating climacteric symptoms in whom even temporary withdrawal of HRT may trigger recurrence of vasomotor and other climacteric symptoms. It is likely that concomitant anticoagulant therapy with warfarin, administered to achieve an INR range of 2.0 to 3.0, will negate any prothrombotic effects of ongoing HRT. This assumption is based on the premise that in patients in whom there is ongoing exposure to a prothrombotic stimulus, such as immobility, warfarin therapy is highly effective in preventing recurrent VTE.[86,87] No prospective studies have assessed the risk of progression of VTE or recurrent disease in women who stop HRT compared with those who continue HRT with concomitant anticoagulant therapy.

Long-Term Management

The optimal duration of anticoagulant therapy is less clear and requires careful consideration of a number of factors. A key issue is whether the episode of VTE occurred during transient exposure to a reversible risk factor for VTE, during exposure to an ongoing risk factor for VTE, or whether the episode was unprovoked (or idiopathic). In patients who develop VTE during exposure to a transient risk factor, such as surgery, three months of treatment is deemed adequate, whereas in patients who develop VTE during exposure to an ongoing risk factor, such as advanced cancer or immobility, indefinite treatment is recommended.[88] The duration of anticoagulant therapy in patients with unprovoked VTE is controversial, although at least three months of treatment is recommended.[88]

The risk of VTE associated with the OC appears to vary with the duration of OC use. Studies suggest that the risk for VTE appears to be highest during the first 6 months to 1 year of OC use, particularly among first-time users.[22,28,34,47,89–92] The risk of VTE diminishes thereafter, but does not disappear during the subsequent years of use.[28] Thus, the OC may be considered a transient and reversible risk factor in women who develop VTE within months of starting the OC, and these patients should be treated for 3 months.[88] However, the argument that the OC is a transient, reversible risk factor is less compelling among women who develop VTE after using the OC for several years. For these patients, the OC may be an "innocent bystander" and not the factor that provoked the thrombotic event. Other factors that confer an ongoing risk for VTE may be present; consequently, anticoagulant therapy for three months may be insufficient to reduce the risk for recurrent VTE. Overall, the duration of anticoagulant therapy should be individualized, as it may be reasonable to treat some patients for only three months whereas other patients may require therapy for 6 months or longer.

The effect of duration of HRT on the risk for VTE has also been studied with similar results as those for the OC. There appears to be a heightened risk during the first year after the start of treatment that diminishes, but does not disappear, during the subsequent four to five years.[6–14] Thus, as discussed previously, the duration of anticoagulant therapy should be individualized with particular attention to the duration of HRT among women who develop VTE. Three months of anticoagulation therapy is reasonable for women who develop VTE within months of starting HRT, whereas women who develop VTE after using HRT for several years may require therapy for 6 months or longer.

KEY LEARNING POINTS

- Clinical studies in different populations and using different designs (case-control, cohort, randomized trial) have established that users of HRT have an approximately two- to threefold increased risk of developing VTE compared with nonusers of HRT, and that users of the OC have an approximately two- to fourfold increased risk of developing VTE compared with nonusers of the OC.

- Use of transdermal (patch) HRT preparations may not be associated with an increased risk for DVT, although additional studies are warranted to further explore this observation.
- In women who are carriers of the factor V Leiden mutation, the risk for VTE is markedly increased with hormone therapy use compared with the risk for VTE in women without the factor V Leiden mutation who do not take hormone therapy.
- Selective screening for thrombophilia may have a role in primary prevention of VTE among women who are seeking to start hormone therapy and for whom there is an increased clinical index of suspicion for a prothrombotic blood disorder.
- Appropriate counseling for women with asymptomatic thrombophilia and no prior VTE who are considering hormone therapy should include a discussion of the variable risks associated with different prothrombotic blood disorders.
- Hormone therapy should generally be avoided in women with symptomatic thrombophilia; however, if used, coadministered antithrombotic therapy with warfarin or LMWH may be a strategy (not formally evaluated) to reduce the risk of recurrent VTE.
- In users of hormone therapy who are undergoing elective surgery and who have no other risk factors for VTE, no compelling evidence exists that hormone therapy needs to be stopped in the perioperative period.
- In contrast, appropriate methods of thromboprophylaxis, which may include temporarily discontinuing hormone therapy before and after surgery, should be considered in patients with other strong risk factors for VTE, such as prior VTE, or anticipated proposed postoperative immobility.
- Initial management of hormone-associated VTE includes stopping the hormone therapy and administering anticoagulant therapy with warfarin (INR range of 2.0–3.0) and unfractionated heparin or LMWH.
- Duration of anticoagulant therapy should be individualized, as three months of therapy may be reasonable among women who develop VTE within months of starting hormone therapy, whereas women who develop VTE after using hormone therapy for several years may require anticoagulation for six months or longer.

REFERENCES

1. United Nations Population Division, Department of Economic and Social Affairs. World contraceptive use 2001. New York: United Nations; 2002.
2. World Health Organization Collaborative Study of Cardiovascular Disease and Steroid Hormone Contraception. Cardiovascular disease and use of oral and injectable progestogen-only contraceptives and combined injectable contraceptives: results of an international, multicenter, case-control study. Contraception 1998;57(5):315–24.
3. Col NF, Weber G, Stiggelbout A, et al. Short-term menopausal hormone therapy for symptom relief. Arch Intern Med 2004;164(15):1634–40.
4. Utian WH, Archer DF, Bachmann DA, et al. Estrogen and progestogen use in postmenopausal women: July 2008 position statement of the North American Menopause Society. Menopause 2008;15(4):584–603.
5. Johnston SL, Farrell SA, Beckerson L, et al. The detection and management of vaginal atrophy. J Obstet Gynaecol Can 2004;26(5):503–8.

6. Daly E, Vessey MP, Hawkins MM, et al. Risk of venous thromboembolism in users of hormone replacement therapy. Lancet 1996;348(9033):977–80.

7. Jick H, Derby LE, Myers MW, et al. Risk of hospital admission for idiopathic venous thromboembolism among users of post-menopausal estrogens. Lancet 1996;348(9033):981–3.

8. Pérez Gutthann S, Garcia Rodriguez LA, Castellsague J, et al. Hormone replacement therapy and risk of venous thromboembolism: population based case-control study. BMJ 1997;314(7083):796–800.

9. Varas-Lorenzo C, García Rodríguez LA, Cattaruzzi C, et al. Hormone replacement therapy and the risk of hospitalization for venous thromboembolism: a population-based study in southern Europe. Am J Epidemiol 1998;147(4):387–90.

10. Grodstein F, Stampfer MJ, Goldhaber SZ, et al. Prospective study of exogenous hormones and risk of pulmonary embolism in women. Lancet 1996;348(9033):983–7.

11. Høibraaten E, Abdelnoor M, Sandset PM. Hormone replacement therapy with estradiol and risk of venous thromboembolism—a population-based case-control study. Thromb Haemost 1999;82(4):1218–21.

12. Douketis JD, Julian JA, Kearon C, et al. Does the type of hormone replacement therapy influence the risk of deep vein thrombosis? A prospective case-control study. J Thromb Haemost 2005;3(5):943–8.

13. Grady D, Wenger NK, Herrington D, et al. Postmenopausal hormone replacement therapy increases risk for venous thromboembolic disease. The Heart and Estrogen/Progestin Replacement Study. Ann Intern Med 2000;132(9):689–96.

14. Writing Group for the Women's Health Initiative Investigators. Risks and benefits of estrogen plus progestin in healthy postmenopausal women. Principal results from the Women's Health Initiative randomized controlled trial. JAMA 2002; 288(3):321–33.

15. Scarabin P-Y, Oger E, Plu-Bureau G, for the Estrogen and ThromboEmbolism Risk (ESTHER) Study Group. Differential association of oral and transdermal oestrogen-replacement therapy with venous thromboembolism risk. Lancet 2003;362(9382):428–32.

16. De Lignieres B, Basdevant A, Thomas G, et al. Biological effects of estradiol-17 beta in postmenopausal women: oral versus percutaneous administration. J Clin Endocrinol Metab 1986;62(3):536–41.

17. Powers MS, Schenkel L, Darley PE, et al. Pharmacokinetics and pharmacodynamics of transdermal dosage forms of 178-estradiol: comparison with conventional oral estrogens used for hormone replacement. Am J Obstet Gynecol 1985;152(8):1099–106.

18. Valla D, Le MG, Poynard T, et al. Risk of hepatic vein thrombosis in relation to recent use of oral contraceptives: a case-control study. Gastroenterology 1986; 90(4):807–11.

19. Thorogood M, Mann J, Murphy M, et al. Risk factors for fatal venous thromboembolism in young women: a case-control study. Int J Epidemiol 1992;21(1):48–52.

20. Quinn DA, Thompson BT, Terrin ML, et al. A prospective investigation of pulmonary embolism in women and men. JAMA 1992;268(13):1689–96.

21. Vandenbroucke JP, Koster T, Briët E, et al. Increased risk of venous thrombosis in oral-contraceptive users who are carriers of factor V Leiden mutation. Lancet 1994;344(8935):1453–7.

22. Spitzer WO, Lewis MA, Heinemann LA, et al. for the Transnational Research Group on Oral Contraceptives and the Health of Young Women. Third generation oral contraceptives and risk of venous thromboembolic disorders: an international case-control study. BMJ 1996;312(7023):83–8.

23. Realini JP, Encarnacion CE, Chintapalli KN, et al. Oral contraceptives and venous thromboembolism: a case-control study designed to minimize detection bias. J Am Board Fam Pract 1997;10(5):315–21.
24. Martinelli I, Sacchi E, Landi G, et al. High risk of cerebral-vein thrombosis in carriers of a prothrombin-gene mutation and in users of oral contraceptives. N Engl J Med 1998;338(25):1793–7.
25. de Bruijn SF, Stam J, Koopman MM, et al. for the Cerebral Venous Sinus Thrombosis Study Group. Case-control study of risk of cerebral sinus thrombosis in oral contraceptive users and in carriers of hereditary prothrombotic conditions. BMJ 1998;316(7131):589–92.
26. Bloemenkamp KW, Rosendaal FR, Büller HR, et al. Risk of venous thrombosis with use of current low-dose oral contraceptives is not explained by diagnostic suspicion and referral bias. Arch Intern Med 1999;159:65–70.
27. Martinelli I, Taioli E, Bucciarelli P, et al. Interaction between the G20210A mutation of the prothrombin gene and oral contraceptive use in deep vein thrombosis. Arterioscler Thromb Vasc Biol 1999;19(3):700–3.
28. Bloemenkamp KW, Rosendaal FR, Helmerhorst FM, et al. Higher risk of venous thrombosis during early use of oral contraceptives in women with inherited clotting defects. Arch Intern Med 2000;160(1):49–52.
29. Parkin L, Skegg DC, Wilson M, et al. Oral contraceptives and fatal pulmonary embolism. Lancet 2000;355(9221):2133–4.
30. Helmrich SP, Rosenberg L, Kaufman DW, et al. Venous thromboembolism in relation to oral contraceptive use. Obstet Gynecol 1987;69(1):91–5.
31. Gerstman BB, Piper JM, Freiman JP, et al. Oral contraceptive oestrogen and progestin potencies and the incidence of deep venous thromboembolism. Int J Epidemiol 1990;19(4):931–6.
32. Hirvonen E, Idänpään-Heikkilä J. Cardiovascular death among women under 40 years of age using low-estrogen oral contraceptives and intrauterine devices in Finland from 1975 to 1984. Am J Obstet Gynecol 1990;163(1 Pt 2):281–4.
33. Gerstman BB, Piper JM, Tomita DK, et al. Oral contraceptive estrogen dose and the risk of deep venous thromboembolic disease. Am J Epidemiol 1991;133(1): 32–7.
34. Poulter NR, Chang CL, Farley TM, et al. for the World Health Organization Collaborative Study of Cardiovascular Disease and Steroid Hormone Contraception Investigators. Venous thromboembolic disease and combined oral contraceptives: results of an international multicentre case-control study. Lancet 1995; 346(8990):1575–82.
35. Jick H, Jick SS, Gurewich V, et al. Risk of idiopathic cardiovascular death and nonfatal venous thromboembolism in women using oral contraceptives with differing progestagen components. Lancet 1995;346(8990):1589–93.
36. Heinemann LA, Lewis MA, Assmann A, et al. Case-control studies on venous thromboembolism: bias due to design? A methodological study on venous thromboembolism and steroid hormone use. Contraception 2002;65(3):207–14.
37. Sartwell PE, Masi AT, Arthes FG, et al. Thromboembolism and oral contraceptives: an epidemiologic case-control study. Am J Epidemiol 1969;90(5): 365–80.
38. Greene GR, Sartwell PE. Oral contraceptive use in patients with thromboembolism following surgery, trauma, or infection. Am J Public Health 1972;62(5):680–5.
39. Oral contraceptives and venous thromboembolic disease, surgically confirmed gallbladder disease, and breast tumours: report from the Boston Collaborative Drug Surveillance Programme. Lancet 1973;1(7817):1399–404.

40. Grounds M. Anovulants: thrombosis and other associated changes. Med J Aust 1974;2(12):440–6.
41. Stolley PD, Tonascia JA, Tockman MS, et al. Thrombosis with low-estrogen oral contraceptives. Am J Epidemiol 1975;102(3):197–208.
42. Maguire MG, Tonascia JA, Sartwell PE, et al. Increased risk of thrombosis due to oral contraceptives: a further report. Am J Epidemiol 1979;110(2):188–95.
43. Petitti DB, Wingerd J, Pellegrin F, et al. Oral contraceptives, smoking, and other factors in relation to risk of venous thromboembolic disease. Am J Epidemiol 1978;108(6):480–5.
44. Petitti DB, Wingerd J, Pellegrin F, et al. Risk of vascular disease in women: smoking, oral contraceptives, noncontraceptive estrogens, and other factors. JAMA 1979;242(11):1150–4.
45. Porter JB, Hunter JR, Jick H, et al. Oral contraceptives and nonfatal vascular disease. Obstet Gynecol 1985;66(1):1–4.
46. Farmer RD, Lawrenson RA, Thompson CR, et al. Population-based study of risk of venous thromboembolism associated with various oral contraceptives. Lancet 1997;349(9045):83–8.
47. Lidegaard Ø, Edstrom B, Kreiner S. Oral contraceptives and venous thromboembolism: a five-year national case-control study. Contraception 2002;65(3):187–96.
48. Vessey MP, Doll R. Investigation of relation between use of oral contraceptives and thromboembolic disease. BMJ 1968;2(5599):199–205.
49. Vessey MP, Doll R. Postoperative thromboembolism and the use of oral contraceptives. BMJ 1970;3(5715):123–6.
50. Bloemenkamp KW, Rosendaal FR, Helmerhorst FM, et al. Enhancement by factor V Leiden mutation of risk of deep-vein thrombosis associated with oral contraceptives containing a third-generation progestagen. Lancet 1995;346(8990):1593–6.
51. Jick H, Kaye JA, Vasilakis-Scaramozza C, et al. Risk of venous thromboembolism among users of third generation oral contraceptives compared with users of oral contraceptives with levonorgestrel before and after 1995: cohort and case-control analysis. BMJ 2000;321(7270):1190–5.
52. Farley TM, Meirik O, Chang CL, et al. for the World Health Organization Collaborative Study of Cardiovascular Disease and Steroid Hormone Contraception Investigators. Effect of different progestagens in low oestrogen oral contraceptives on venous thromboembolic disease. Lancet 1995;346(8990):1582–8.
53. Lidegaard Ø, Edström B, Kreiner S. Oral contraceptives and venous thromboembolism: a case-control study. Contraception 1998;57(5):291–301.
54. Andersen BS, Olsen J, Nielsen GL, et al. Third generation oral contraceptives and heritable thrombophilia as risk factors of non-fatal venous thromboembolism. Thromb Haemost 1998;79(1):23–31.
55. Farmer RD, Todd J-C, Lewis MA, et al. The risks of venous thromboembolic disease among German women using oral contraceptives: a database study. Contraception 1998;57(2):67–70.
56. Herings RM, Urquhart J, Leufkens HG. Venous thromboembolism among new users of different oral contraceptives. Lancet 1999;354(9173):127–8 [erratum appears in: Lancet 1999;354:1478].
57. Burnhill MS. The use of a large-scale surveillance system in Planned Parenthood Federation of America Clinics to monitor cardiovascular events in users of combination oral contraceptives. Int J Fertil Womens Med 1999;44(1):19–30.

58. Farmer RD, Lawrenson RA, Todd J-C, et al. A comparison of the risks of venous thromboembolic disease in association with different combined oral contraceptives. Br J Clin Pharmacol 2000;49(6):580–90.

59. Oral contraceptives, venous thrombosis, and varicose veins: Royal College of General Practitioners' Oral Contraception Study. J R Coll Gen Pract 1978; 28(192):393–9.

60. Porter JB, Hunter JR, Danielson DA, et al. Oral contraceptives and nonfatal vascular disease: recent experience. Obstet Gynecol 1982;59(3):299–302.

61. Vessey M, Mant D, Smith A, et al. Oral contraceptives and venous thromboembolism: findings in a large prospective study. Br Med J (Clin Res Ed) 1986; 292(6519):526.

62. Fuertes-de la Haba A, Curet JO, Pelegrina I, et al. Thrombophlebitis among oral and nonoral contraceptive users. Obstet Gynecol 1971;38(2):259–63.

63. Vandenbroucke JP, van der Meer FJ, Helmerhorst FM, et al. Factor V Leiden: should we screen oral contraceptive users and pregnant women? BMJ 1996; 313(7065):1127–30.

64. McColl MD, Ramsay JE, Tait RC, et al. Risk factors for pregnancy associated venous thromboembolism. Thromb Haemost 1997;78(4):1183–8.

65. Lindqvist P, Dahlback B, Marsal K. Thrombotic risk during pregnancy: a population study. Obstet Gynecol 1999;94(4):595–9.

66. Pabinger I, Schneider B, for the GTH Study Group on Natural Inhibitors. Thrombotic risk of women with hereditary antithrombin III-, protein C- and protein S-deficiency taking oral contraceptive medication. Thromb Haemost 1994;71(5): 548–52.

67. Gomes MP, Deitcher SR. Risk of venous thromboembolic disease associated with hormonal contraceptives and hormone replacement therapy: a clinical review. Arch Intern Med 2004;164(18):1965–76.

68. Mattsson LA, Cullberg G. Vaginal absorption of two estriol preparations. A comparative study in postmenopausal women. Acta Obstet Gynecol Scand 1983;62(5):393–6.

69. Iosif CS. Effects of protracted administration of estriol on the lower genitourinary tract in postmenopausal women. Arch Gynecol Obstet 1992;251(3): 115–20.

70. Henriksson L, Stjernquist M, Boquist L, et al. A one year multicenter study of efficacy and safety of a continuous, low-dose, estradiol-releasing vaginal ring (Estring) in postmenopausal women with symptoms and signs of urogenital aging. Am J Obstet Gynecol 1996;174(1 Pt 1):85–92.

71. Rioux JE, Devlin C, Gelfand MM, et al. 17-β-Estradiol vaginal tablets versus conjugated equine estrogen cream to relieve menopausal atrophic vaginitis. Menopause 2000;7(3):156–61.

72. Mettler L, Olsen PG. Long-term treatment of atrophic vaginitis with low-dose oestradiol vaginal tablets. Maturitas 1991;14(1):23–31.

73. Mattsson LA, Cullberg G, Eriksson O, et al. Vaginal administration of low-dose oestradiol—effects on the endometrium and vaginal cytology. Maturitas 1989; 11(3):217–22.

74. Rosing J, Middeldorp S, Curvers J, et al. Low-dose oral contraceptives and acquired resistance to activated protein C: a randomized cross-over study. Lancet 1999;354(9195):2036–40.

75. Kemmeren JM, Algra A, Grobbee DE. Third generation oral contraceptives and risk of venous thrombosis: meta-analysis. BMJ 2001;323(7305):1–9.

76. Hirsh J, Baner KA, Donati MB, et al. Parenteral anticongulants: American College of Chest Physicians Evidence based Practice guidelines (8th edition). Chest 2008;133(6):141S–59S.

77. Cushman M, Kuller LH, Prentice R, et al. Estrogen plus progestin and risk of venous thrombosis. JAMA 2004;292:1573–80.

78. Canonico M, Plu-Bureau G, Lowe GD, et al. Hormone replacement therapy and risk of venous thromboembolism in postmenopausal women: systematic review and meta-analysis. BMJ 2008;336(2):1227–31.

79. Stratzec C, Oger T, Yon de Jonge-Cononico MB, et al. Prothrombotic mutations, hormone therapy, and venous thromboembolism among postmenopausal women: impact of the route of estrogen administration. Circulation 2005;112: 3495–500.

80. Crowther MA, Keltan JG. Congenital thrombophilia states associated with venous thrombosis: a qualitative review and proposed classification system. Ann Intern Med 2003;138:128–34.

81. Wallace WA. HRT and the surgeon. Guidelines from the Royal College of Surgeons of Edinburgh. J R Coll Surg Edinb 1993;38(2):58–61.

82. Ardern DW, Atkinson DR, Fenton AJ. Peri-operative use of oestrogen containing medications and deep vein thrombosis: a national survey. N Z Med J 2002; 115(1157):U26.

83. Geerts WH, Pineo GF, Heit HA, et al. Prevention of venous thromboembolism. American College of Chest Physicians Evidence based clinical practice guidelines (8th edition). Chest 2008;133(6):381S–453S.

84. Hurbaneck JG, Jaffer AK, Morra N, et al. Postmenopausal hormone replacement and venous thromboembolism following hip and knee arthroplasty. Thromb Haemost 2004;92(2):337–43.

85. Douketis JD, Julian JA, Costantini L, et al. HRT-DVT Study Group. HRT and the risk of DVT: the role of progesterone and other factors in the pathogenesis of HRT-associated DVT. Thromb Haemost 2001;86(Suppl 1):OC850.

86. Kearon C. Duration of therapy for acute venous thromboembolism. Clin Chest Med 2003;24(1):63–72.

87. Rosendaal FR. Venous thrombosis: a multicausal disease. Lancet 1999; 353(9159):1167–73.

88. Keaon C, Kahn SR, Agnelli G, et al. Antithrombotic therapy for venous thromboembolic disease: American College of Chest Physician Evidence-based Clinical Practice guideline (8th edition). Chest 2008;133(6):454S–545S.

89. Bottinger LE, Westerholm B. Oral contraceptives and thromboembolic disease. Swedish experience. Acta Med Scand 1971;190(5):455–63.

90. Suissa S, Blais L, Spitzer WO, et al. First-time use of newer oral contraceptives and the risk of venous thromboembolism. Contraception 1997;56(3):141–6.

91. Farley TM, Meirik O, Marmot MG, et al. Oral contraceptives and risk of venous thromboembolism: impact of duration of use. Contraception 1998;57(1):61–5.

92. Poulter NR, Farley TM, Chang CL, et al. Safety of combined oral contraceptive pills. Lancet 1996;347(9000):547.

Cancer-Associated Thrombosis

John Winters, MD[a], David Garcia, MD[b],*

KEYWORDS

- Cancer • Venous thromboembolism • Pathology • Prophylaxis
- Treatment • Central-venous catheter(s)

The pathophysiology of the prothrombotic state of cancer is complex and multifactorial, resulting from a detrimental combination of intrinsic tumor cell properties, therapeutic interventions, and prolonged severe illness, which promote venous thromboembolic events through direct interactions with coagulation pathways, venous stasis, and endothelial injury (**Fig. 1**). Investigators have identified many possible molecular explanations by which tumor cells might affect the coagulant potential of the blood, such as increased levels of inflammatory cytokines (eg, tumor necrosis factor α and interleukin-1) and oncogene-mediated alterations in the levels of important proteins such as plasminogen activator inhibitor 1 (PAI-1). Three of the most studied candidates (tissue factor, cancer procoagulant, and mucin) are discussed here.

Tissue factor (TF), a transmembrane glycoprotein, is the primary cellular initiator of the extrinsic coagulation pathway, and is most notably expressed on the surface of subendothelial cells, platelets, and cell-derived microparticles. Tumor cells in a wide variety of malignancies overexpress TF on their surface and in association with microparticles; increased expression of TF appears to be associated with a significantly increased incidence of thrombotic events.[1–6] In one study of 41 patients with pancreatic cancer, immunohistochemical staining showed that higher TF expression was associated with venous thromboembolism (VTE) (odds ratio, 4.5).[4]

Cancer procoagulant (CP) is a 68-kDa vitamin K–dependent protein found exclusively in amniotic-chorionic tissues and malignant cells.[7,8] In ex vivo studies, CP directly activates factor X in the absence of factor VII and has been shown to activate platelets with a mechanism similar to thrombin.[9,10] CP has been identified in the serum of 85% of cancer patients.[11]

[a] Department of Internal Medicine, University of New Mexico School of Medicine, MSC01-5550, 1 University of New Mexico, Albuquerque, NM 87131, USA
[b] Division of Hematology and Oncology, Department of Internal Medicine, University of New Mexico School of Medicine, MSC07-4025, 1 University of New Mexico, Albuquerque, NM 87131, USA
* Corresponding author.
E-mail address: DAVGarcia@salud.unm.edu

Hematol Oncol Clin N Am 24 (2010) 695–707
doi:10.1016/j.hoc.2010.05.004
0889-8588/10/$ – see front matter © 2010 Elsevier Inc. All rights reserved.

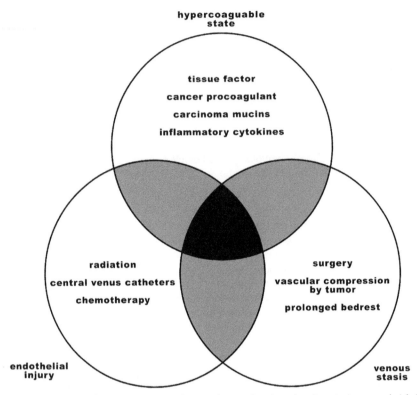

Fig. 1. Mechanisms of cancer-associated VTE. The mechanisms leading to increased risk for VTE in cancer patients are multifactorial, complex, and cumulative.

The increased risk of thrombotic events associated with mucinous adenocarcinoma is well known. This phenomenon may in part result from the emission of abnormal mucins into the circulation; mucins interact with leukocytes and platelets through circulating L- and P-selectin molecules. These interactions lead to the activation of platelets, causing the formation of thrombi.[12,13]

In addition to the cellular mechanisms described in the preceding paragraphs, multiple extrinsic factors contribute to increased risk of venous thromboembolic events in cancer patients. For example, chemotherapy, radiation, surgery, direct compression of a blood vessel by a bulky tumor, immobilization, and placement of central venous catheters can all play a role in the formation of a pathologic clot.[14–18] Although a number of chemotherapy agents predispose to thrombosis, anti-angiogenic drugs such as thalidomide (Thalomid), lenalidomide (Revlimid), and beva-cizumab (Avastin) may pose an especially high risk for patients who receive them in combination with corticosteroids or additional chemotherapy.[19–21] Recently, erythropoiesis-stimulating agents such as epoetin (Epogen, Procrit) and darbopoetin (Aranesp) have also been associated with malignancy-associated VTE.[22]

PRIMARY PREVENTION OF VENOUS THROMBOEMBOLISM IN CANCER PATIENTS

In selected, high-risk cancer patients, thromboprophylaxis has the potential to improve outcomes. Hospitalization increases the risk of VTE in cancer patients.[23]

Multiple large, randomized controlled studies have found that use of low-molecular-weight heparins (LMWH) or fondaparinux (Arixtra) significantly reduces the incidence of VTE in patients hospitalized for acute medical illness without increasing the incidence of adverse events compared with placebo.[24–26] A meta-analysis of multiple randomized controlled trials (RCTs) enrolling a heterogeneous group of "medically ill" inpatients suggests that unfractionated heparin (UFH) has efficacy and safety profiles comparable to LMWH.[27] Unfortunately, no studies of VTE prevention specifically in cancer patients admitted for medical reasons have been performed.

Both the American Society of Clinical Oncology (ASCO) and the American College of Chest Physicians (ACCP) recommend that hospitalized cancer patients be considered as candidates for pharmacologic VTE prophylaxis in the absence of bleeding or other contraindications.[28–30] Provider compliance with thromboprophylaxis guidelines is particularly low in cancer patients,[31,32] perhaps because thrombocytopenia and other bleeding risk factors are common in these patients. The platelet count below which the risk of "prophylactic-dose" heparin or LMWH outweighs the benefit is not known. Institution-based alert systems may increase physician compliance with pharmacologic prophylaxis, and reduce the incidence of deep venous thrombosis (DVT) and pulmonary embolism (PE) in hospitalized patients.[33,34]

The utility of thromboprophylaxis in ambulatory cancer patients has been investigated in multiple clinical trials.[35–39] A recent trial randomized 1150 ambulatory patients with metastatic or locally advanced cancer to receive thromboprophylaxis with nadroparin (Fraxiparine) versus placebo while undergoing treatment with chemotherapy. A significant reduction in VTE was observed (from 3.9% to 2.0%), although the overall effect was small (absolute risk reduction 1.9%; number needed to treat 52.6).[35] Interim analysis of 2 RCTs investigating chemoprophylaxis with LMWH in patients with advanced pancreatic cancer receiving chemotherapy demonstrated a significant decrease in the rate of both VTE and death in this population.[38,39] Current practice guidelines do not recommend the use of thromboprophylaxis for ambulatory cancer patients, with the exception of those undergoing treatment with thalidomide or lenalidomide in combination with high-dose steroids or chemotherapy.[29]

Although studies support the use of pharmacologic prophylaxis in patients with cancer, the unanswered question is: in which patients can the risk and inconvenience of primary VTE prophylaxis be justified? The identification of such a subgroup will be difficult in clinical practice, but a risk-stratification model developed by Khorana and colleagues (for chemotherapy-associated thrombosis) may be helpful; the model uses readily available clinical and laboratory data to divide patients into groups at low, intermediate, or high risk for VTE. The high-risk group developed symptomatic VTE at a rate of approximately 6.7% over a median time of 2.5 months.[40] This was much higher than the 0.3% of patients in the low-risk group who developed VTE (**Fig. 2**).

Compared with patients without cancer who undergo major surgery, cancer patients are at increased risk (both magnitude and duration) of developing postoperative venous thromboembolic events. VTE is the most common cause of death during the first 30 days after major oncologic surgeries.[41,42] Advanced age, late-stage malignancy, prolonged anesthesia, protracted time of immobilization, and prior history of VTE are associated with increased risk of postsurgical VTE.[41]

Well-designed trials have shown that LMWH and UFH effectively reduce the incidence of VTE in patients undergoing major abdominal or pelvic surgery for malignancy without increasing the risk of adverse events.[43–45] A systematic review and meta-analysis of 14 RCTs involving 3986 patients with cancer found no differences in mortality when using LMWH versus UFH for perioperative thromboprophylaxis.[46]

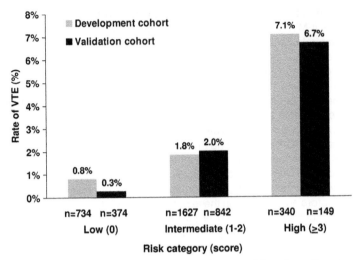

Fig. 2. Rates of VTE among ambulatory cancer patients receiving chemotherapy, according to scores from the risk model in the derivation and validation cohorts. (*From* Khorana AA, Kuderer NM, Culakova E, et al. Development and validation of a predictive model for chemotherapy-associated thrombosis. Blood 2008;111(10):4902–7; with permission.)

Although definitive evidence is not yet available, at least 2 studies have found that higher doses of LMWH are more efficacious and equally safe for preventing VTE when compared with lower doses of LMWH in surgical cancer patients.[47,48] A randomized controlled trial in patients undergoing high-risk abdominal surgery found fondaparinux to have equal efficacy and safety when compared with dalteparin for VTE prophylaxis. Post hoc analysis of patients with cancer revealed possible superior efficacy of fondaparinux in this subpopulation but this finding needs confirmation in a prospective trial.[49] Consensus guidelines recommend UFH, fondaparinux, or LMWH as VTE prophylaxis for cancer patients undergoing major surgery.[29,30]

The results of more than one clinical trial indicate that prolonged use of LMWH (4 weeks) compared with short-term use (1 week) for thromboprophylaxis in patients who have undergone pelvic or abdominal surgery for cancer reduces the risk of venographically detected VTE, and does not carry an increased risk of bleeding or adverse events.[50,51] Although a recent systematic review highlights the need for more evidence of net benefit, both the ACCP and ASCO guidelines suggest 4 weeks of LMWH (extending past the period of hospitalization) for "higher risk" patients.[29,30,52]

Neurosurgical interventions in patients with cancer are associated with high rates of venous thromboembolic events. Pharmacologic prophylaxis has traditionally been avoided in these patients because of concerns about intracranial bleeding.[53] A small RCT found that postoperative LMWH combined with graduated compression stockings significantly decreases the incidence of VTE when compared with compression stockings alone, without increasing the risk of intracranial bleeding.[54] The ACCP guidelines recommend UFH or LMWH combined with mechanical prophylaxis in all high-risk neurosurgery patients.[30]

Gynecologic surgery for malignancy also carries a considerable risk for thromboembolic complications. Studies have shown that UFH significantly reduces DVT in this group of patients, when compared with no prophylaxis, and that LMWH has a similar efficacy and safety profile to UFH in this group.[55–57] The ACCP recommends UFH or

LMWH, combined with mechanical prophylaxis, in all patients undergoing surgery for gynecologic malignancy, and 4 weeks of LMWH extended past the hospitalization for higher risk patients.[30]

TREATMENT OF VTE IN CANCER

Pharmacologic anticoagulation is highly effective in preventing complications of VTE as well as recurrent events. A strategy of initial anticoagulation with LMWH, fondaparinux, or intravenous (IV) UFH followed by long-term targeted therapy with an oral vitamin K antagonist (VKA) is widely used to treat acute VTE in the general population. However, the long-term use of oral VKAs in cancer patients is less effective and less safe when compared with patients without cancer.[28,58] For the initial treatment of VTE, LMWH is preferred in cancer patients because it can be used in an outpatient setting, does not require laboratory monitoring, and has a lower risk of heparin-induced thrombocytopenia.[59–64] Furthermore, a recent systematic review suggests that LMWH may be more effective than UFH in this setting.[65] The efficacy of fondaparinux is comparable to heparin or LMWH in initial treatment of VTE for patients without cancer;[60,61] however, there is a lack of cancer-specific evidence to support its use for the treatment of malignancy-associated VTE.

The largest RCT comparing long-term treatment (ie, secondary prevention) of VTE in cancer patients found LMWH was more efficacious and had a similar rate of bleeding complications when compared with a VKA. A total of 672 patients were randomized to receive monotherapy with dalteparin, or dalteparin followed by a coumarin for 6 months. Twenty-seven (9%) of 336 patients who received monotherapy with dalteparin had a recurrent VTE at 6 months compared with 53 (17%) of 336 patients in the control group, a relative risk reduction of 52%.[66] Compared with VKA treatment, the risk of major bleeding was not increased by long-term therapy with LMWH. A recent Cochrane Collaboration systematic review confirmed the superiority of LMWH compared with VKAs in the secondary prevention of VTE in cancer patients.[67] Practice guidelines produced by the ACCP, National Cancer Center Network (NCCN), and ASCO recommend treatment with LMWH for 3 to 6 months following initial VTE and indefinitely if active cancer or other risk factors persist.[29,68,69]

VTE (usually pulmonary embolism) may present in an otherwise asymptomatic cancer patient as an incidental finding on routine imaging; the prevalence of these unsuspected thrombi is 1.9% to 6.3% in patients undergoing CT scan for staging purposes.[70,71] A recent retrospective-cohort study compared mortality in 104 cancer patients with symptomatic VTE, 37 cancer patients with asymptomatic VTE, and 48 cancer patients with no VTE. All patients with symptomatic or asymptomatic VTE received anticoagulation with UFH or LMWH. Six-month mortality in the groups with symptomatic and asymptomatic VTE was similar (48.6% and 51.0%) and was significantly higher than the group with no VTE (27.1%).[72] Although the impact of anticoagulant therapy on mortality or VTE recurrence risk in cancer patients who have asymptomatic VTE is unknown, ACCP practice guidelines recommend therapeutic anticoagulation comparable to what would be used for cancer patients whose VTE is symptomatic.[69]

Inferior vena cava (IVC) filters have a limited role in the treatment of cancer-associated VTE. When added to anticoagulation therapy in VTE patients without cancer, placement of permanent IVC filters reduces the incidence PE from 15.1% to 6.2%; however, the incidence of DVT increases and there is no overall survival benefit at 8 years.[73] Evidence from cancer-specific studies investigating use of permanent or retrievable IVC filters for treatment of VTE is lacking. IVC filter placement is appropriate for cancer patients with symptomatic VTE who have contraindications to anticoagulation.[29,68]

CENTRAL VENOUS CATHETER–RELATED THROMBOSIS IN CANCER PATIENTS

Central venous catheters (CVC) are commonly used in cancer patients. Infection and VTE complicate their use. The incidence of catheter-related thrombosis in cancer patients is variable; in the largest prospective study to date, 4.3% of patients developed symptomatic CVC-associated DVT.[15,74,75] Upper extremity DVTs associated with CVC can result in significant morbidity and mortality. Monreal and colleagues[76] prospectively observed 86 non–CVC-associated upper extremity DVTs in patients who did not have cancer: 13 patients were diagnosed with PE, and 2 died from PE despite adequate therapy with intravenous heparin. Another prospective study followed 53 patients with upper extremity DVT who did not have cancer, 27.3% of whom developed post-thrombotic syndrome at 2 years.[77] CVC-related thrombosis usually develops in the ipsilateral subclavian vein, innominate vein, or rarely the superior vena cava within 4 to 8 weeks following placement of a central venous catheter. It may occur less frequently with tip placement at the junction of the superior vena cava and the right atrium.[74,75]

The use of anticoagulation for thromboprophylaxis in patients with long-term indwelling catheters has been investigated in multiple RCTs; meta-analyses and systematic reviews of the available evidence yield conflicting results.[78–85] A recent meta-analysis of 9 randomized, prospective trials evaluated the efficacy of thromboprophylaxis in patients with cancer. Data from 852 patients who received heparin (UFH or LMWH) showed a nonsignificant reduction of symptomatic DVT (relative risk [RR], 0.43; 95% confidence interval [CI], 0.18–1.08), with no effect on mortality (RR, 0.74; 95% CI, 0.40–1.36) or major bleeding (RR, 0.68; 95% CI, 0.10–4.78). In the 1007 patients who received warfarin (or no treatment), no statistically significant impact on the risk of CVC-associated thrombosis was seen (RR, 0.62; 95% CI, 0.30–1.27).[83] Current ACCP, NCCN, and ASCO guidelines do not recommend routine thromboprophylaxis in cancer patients with indwelling CVCs.[29,30,68]

There is insufficient evidence to make strong recommendations about the treatment of catheter-related thrombosis in cancer patients. In one nonrandomized, prospective study, 46 patients (34 with cancer) with upper extremity DVT were anticoagulated with dalteparin for a minimum of 5 days, followed by long-term targeted warfarin therapy (international normalized ratio [INR]: 2.0–3.0). At 12 weeks, 1 patient had recurrence of DVT and 1 patient had a significant bleed.[86] ACCP recommendations for treatment of upper extremity DVT are similar to guidelines for treating lower extremity DVTs, as no large randomized trials have compared efficacy, intensity, or duration of therapy with patients in this population. In response to the lack of expert recommendations addressing the treatment of catheter-related thrombosis in cancer patients, a multidisciplinary working group established by the French National Federation of Cancer Centers recently published guidelines according to the Standards, Options, and Recommendations methodology (SOR). The SOR guidelines recommend treating CVC-associated thrombosis in cancer patients with prolonged use of LMWH, and that long-term anticoagulation with a VKA should be reserved for patients with severe renal impairment.[87]

Removal of the catheter in patients with CVC-associated upper extremity DVT should be considered but is not obligatory. The benefit of line removal was examined (along with other treatment modalities) in a retrospective study involving 319 cancer patients, of whom 112 had CVC-related thrombosis identified with radionucleotide imaging. All patients received one or more of the following interventions: warfarin, line removal, or line replacement. Regardless of the intervention, no major complications such as PE or death occurred. All patients in the study, except 4 who had been treated with line replacement, had complete resolution of their presenting symptoms.[16] Another clinical trial treated 74 patients with active malignancy and CVC-associated upper extremity thrombosis with dalteparin and warfarin. After 3 months of treatment, no patients had recurrence of VTE, and no CVCs had been removed because of line failure or VTE recurrence/extension.[88] The most recent guideline published by the ACCP does not recommend removal of an indwelling catheter if the device is functioning, and there is an ongoing need for the catheter.[30] The SOR guidelines state that maintenance of the catheter is justified in the event that the catheter is mandatory, functional, in the right position, not infected, and showing a favorable evolution under close monitoring.[87]

SUMMARY

Venous thromboembolic events in cancer patients cause significant morbidity and mortality. Basic science and clinical investigations are needed to broaden our understanding of their underlying pathophysiology, as well as to optimize prevention and treatment strategies. Emerging data will identify high-risk subgroups that will derive significant net benefit from primary prophylaxis against VTE. The treatment of VTE in cancer patients is more complex than in patients without cancer. Such patients have worse outcomes and the risk:benefit ratios of anticoagulants vary compared with patients who do not have cancer. Long-term treatment with LMWH is superior to oral VKAs when treating VTE in the setting of malignancy and should be prescribed in the absence of contraindications or other barriers to LMWH use. As the understanding of cancer-associated VTE evolves, recommendations and guidelines are expected to change frequently.

REFERENCES

1. Tesselaar ME, Romijn FP, Van Der Linden IK, et al. Microparticle-associated tissue factor activity: a link between cancer and thrombosis? J Thromb Haemost 2007;5(3):520–7.
2. Davila M, Amirkhosravi A, Coll E, et al. Tissue factor-bearing microparticles derived from tumor cells: impact on coagulation activation. J Thromb Haemost 2008;6(9):1517–24.
3. Tesselaar ME, Romijn FP, van der Linden IK, et al. Microparticle-associated tissue factor activity in cancer patients with and without thrombosis. J Thromb Haemost 2009;7(8):1421–3.
4. Khorana AA, Ahrendt SA, Ryan CK, et al. Tissue factor expression, angiogenesis, and thrombosis in pancreatic cancer. Clin Cancer Res 2007;13(10):2870–5.
5. Uno K, Homma S, Satoh T, et al. Tissue factor expression as a possible determinant of thromboembolism in ovarian cancer. Br J Cancer 2007;96(2):290–5.
6. Khorana AA, Francis CW, Menzies KE, et al. Plasma tissue factor may be predictive of venous thromboembolism in pancreatic cancer. J Thromb Haemost 2008; 6(11):1983–5.
7. Donati MB, Gambacorti-Passerini C, Casali B, et al. Cancer procoagulant in human tumor cells: evidence from melanoma patients. Cancer Res 1986;46(12 Pt 1):6471–4.
8. Gordon SG, Hasiba U, Cross BA, et al. Cysteine proteinase procoagulant from amnion-chorion. Blood 1985;66(6):1261–5.

9. Falanga A, Gordon SG. Isolation and characterization of cancer procoagulant: a cysteine proteinase from malignant tissue. Biochemistry 1985;24(20):5558–67.

10. Olas B, Wachowicz B, Mielicki WP. Role of phosphoinositide 3-kinase in adhesion of platelets to fibrinogen stimulated by cancer procoagulant. Platelets 2001; 12(7):431–5.

11. Gordon SG, Cross BA. An enzyme-linked immunosorbent assay for cancer procoagulant and its potential as a new tumor marker. Cancer Res 1990;50(19): 6229–34.

12. Kim YJ, Borsig L, Han HL, et al. Distinct selectin ligands on colon carcinoma mucins can mediate pathological interactions among platelets, leukocytes, and endothelium. Am J Pathol 1999;155(2):461–72.

13. Wahrenbrock M, Borsig L, Le D, et al. Selectin-mucin interactions as a probable molecular explanation for the association of Trousseau syndrome with mucinous adenocarcinomas. J Clin Invest 2003;112(6):853–62.

14. Otten HM, Mathijssen J, ten Cate H, et al. Symptomatic venous thromboembolism in cancer patients treated with chemotherapy: an underestimated phenomenon. Arch Intern Med 2004;164(2):190–4.

15. Lee AY, Levine MN, Butler G, et al. Incidence, risk factors, and outcomes of catheter-related thrombosis in adult patients with cancer. J Clin Oncol 2006; 24(9):1404–8.

16. Frank DA, Meuse J, Hirsch D, et al. The treatment and outcome of cancer patients with thromboses on central venous catheters. J Thromb Thrombolysis 2000;10(3): 271–5.

17. Blom JW, Vanderschoot JP, Oostindier MJ, et al. Incidence of venous thrombosis in a large cohort of 66,329 cancer patients: results of a record linkage study. J Thromb Haemost 2006;4(3):529–35.

18. Heit JA, Silverstein MD, Mohr DN, et al. Risk factors for deep vein thrombosis and pulmonary embolism: a population-based case-control study. Arch Intern Med 2000;160(6):809–15.

19. Zangari M, Anaissie E, Barlogie B, et al. Increased risk of deep-vein thrombosis in patients with multiple myeloma receiving thalidomide and chemotherapy. Blood 2001;98(5):1614–5.

20. Menon SP, Rajkumar SV, Lacy M, et al. Thromboembolic events with lenalidomide-based therapy for multiple myeloma. Cancer 2008;112(7): 1522–8.

21. Scappaticci FA, Skillings JR, Holden SN, et al. Arterial thromboembolic events in patients with metastatic carcinoma treated with chemotherapy and bevacizumab. J Natl Cancer Inst 2007;99(16):1232–9.

22. Bohlius J, Wilson J, Seidenfeld J, et al. Recombinant human erythropoietins and cancer patients: updated meta-analysis of 57 studies including 9353 patients. J Natl Cancer Inst 2006;98(10):708–14.

23. Kroger K, Weiland D, Ose C, et al. Risk factors for venous thromboembolic events in cancer patients. Ann Oncol 2006;17(2):297–303.

24. Cohen AT, Davidson BL, Gallus AS, et al. Efficacy and safety of fondaparinux for the prevention of venous thromboembolism in older acute medical patients: randomised placebo controlled trial. BMJ 2006;332(7537):325–9.

25. Leizorovicz A, Cohen AT, Turpie AG, et al. Randomized, placebo-controlled trial of dalteparin for the prevention of venous thromboembolism in acutely ill medical patients. Circulation 2004;110(7):874–9.

26. Samama MM, Cohen AT, Darmon JY, et al. A comparison of enoxaparin with placebo for the prevention of venous thromboembolism in acutely ill medical

patients. Prophylaxis in medical patients with Enoxaparin Study Group. N Engl J Med 1999;341(11):793–800.

27. Mismetti P, Laporte-Simitsidis S, Tardy B, et al. Prevention of venous thromboembolism in internal medicine with unfractionated or low-molecular-weight heparins: a meta-analysis of randomised clinical trials. Thromb Haemost 2000;83(1):14–9.

28. Prandoni P, Lensing AW, Piccioli A, et al. Recurrent venous thromboembolism and bleeding complications during anticoagulant treatment in patients with cancer and venous thrombosis. Blood 2002;100(10):3484–8.

29. Lyman GH, Khorana AA, Falanga A, et al. American Society of Clinical Oncology guideline: recommendations for venous thromboembolism prophylaxis and treatment in patients with cancer. J Clin Oncol 2007;25(34):5490–505.

30. Geerts WH, Bergqvist D, Pineo GF, et al. Prevention of venous thromboembolism: American College of Chest Physicians evidence-based clinical practice guidelines (8th edition). Chest 2008;133(Suppl 6):381S–453S.

31. Cohen AT, Tapson VF, Bergmann JF, et al. Venous thromboembolism risk and prophylaxis in the acute hospital care setting (ENDORSE study): a multinational cross-sectional study. Lancet 2008;371(9610):387–94.

32. Amin A, Stemkowski S, Lin J, et al. Thromboprophylaxis rates in US medical centers: success or failure? J Thromb Haemost 2007;5(8):1610–6.

33. Kucher N, Koo S, Quiroz R, et al. Electronic alerts to prevent venous thromboembolism among hospitalized patients. N Engl J Med 2005;352(10):969–77.

34. Garcia DA, Highfill J, Finnerty K, et al. A prospective, controlled trial of a pharmacy-driven alert system to increase thromboprophylaxis rates in medical inpatients. Blood Coagul Fibrinolysis 2009;20(7):541–5.

35. Agnelli G, Gussoni G, Bianchini C, et al. Nadroparin for the prevention of thromboembolic events in ambulatory patients with metastatic or locally advanced solid cancer receiving chemotherapy: a randomised, placebo-controlled, double-blind study. Lancet Oncol 2009;10(10):943–9.

36. Levine M, Hirsh J, Gent M, et al. Double-blind randomised trial of a very-low-dose warfarin for prevention of thromboembolism in stage IV breast cancer. Lancet 1994;343(8902):886–9.

37. Perry JR, Rogers L, Laperriere N, et al. PRODIGE: a phase III randomized placebo-controlled trial of thromboprophylaxis using dalteparin low molecular weight heparin (LMWH) in patients with newly diagnosed malignant glioma [abstract 2011]. J Clin Oncol 2007;25(Pt 1):18s. 43rd ASCO Annual Meeting Proceedings, Chicago.

38. Maraveyas A, Holmes M, Lofts F, et al. Chemoanticoagulation versus chemotherapy in advanced pancreatic cancer (APC): results of the interim analysis of the FRAGEM trial [abstract 4583]. J Clin Oncol 2007;25(Pt 1):18s. 43rd ASCO Annual Meeting Proceedings, Chicago.

39. Riess H, Pelzer U, Deutschinoff G, et al. A prospective, randomized trial of chemotherapy with or without the low-molecular weight heparin (LMWH) enoxaparin in patients (pts) with advanced pancreatic cancer (APC): results of the CONKO-004 trial [abstract 4506]. J Clin Oncol 2009;27(Pt 1):18s. 45th Annual Meeting Proceedings, Orlando.

40. Khorana AA, Kuderer NM, Culakova E, et al. Development and validation of a predictive model for chemotherapy-associated thrombosis. Blood 2008;111(10):4902–7.

41. Agnelli G, Bolis G, Capussotti L, et al. A clinical outcome-based prospective study on venous thromboembolism after cancer surgery: the @RISTOS project. Ann Surg 2006;243(1):89–95.

42. Rickles FR, Levine MN. Epidemiology of thrombosis in cancer. Acta Haematol 2001;106(1–2):6–12.

43. Fricker JP, Vergnes Y, Schach R, et al. Low dose heparin versus low molecular weight heparin (Kabi 2165, Fragmin) in the prophylaxis of thromboembolic complications of abdominal oncological surgery. Eur J Clin Invest 1988;18(6): 561–7.

44. Efficacy and safety of enoxaparin versus unfractionated heparin for prevention of deep vein thrombosis in elective cancer surgery: a double-blind randomized multicentre trial with venographic assessment. ENOXACAN Study Group. Br J Surg 1997;84(8):1099–103.

45. McLeod RS, Geerts WH, Sniderman KW, et al. Subcutaneous heparin versus low-molecular-weight heparin as thromboprophylaxis in patients undergoing colorectal surgery: results of the Canadian colorectal DVT prophylaxis trial: a randomized, double-blind trial. Ann Surg 2001;233(3):438–44.

46. Akl EA, Terrenato I, Barba M, et al. Low-molecular-weight heparin vs unfractionated heparin for perioperative thromboprophylaxis in patients with cancer: a systematic review and meta-analysis. Arch Intern Med 2008;168(12):1261–9.

47. Bergqvist D, Burmark US, Flordal PA, et al. Low molecular weight heparin started before surgery as prophylaxis against deep vein thrombosis: 2500 versus 5000 XaI units in 2070 patients. Br J Surg 1995;82(4):496–501.

48. Balibrea JL, Altimiras J, Larruzea I, et al. Optimal dosing of bemiparin as prophylaxis against venous thromboembolism in surgery for cancer: an audit of practice. Int J Surg 2007;5(2):114–9.

49. Agnelli G, Bergqvist D, Cohen AT, et al. Randomized clinical trial of postoperative fondaparinux versus perioperative dalteparin for prevention of venous thromboembolism in high-risk abdominal surgery. Br J Surg 2005;92(10):1212–20.

50. Rasmussen MS, Jorgensen LN, Wille-Jorgensen P, et al. Prolonged prophylaxis with dalteparin to prevent late thromboembolic complications in patients undergoing major abdominal surgery: a multicenter randomized open-label study. J Thromb Haemost 2006;4(11):2384–90.

51. Bergqvist D, Agnelli G, Cohen AT, et al. Duration of prophylaxis against venous thromboembolism with enoxaparin after surgery for cancer. N Engl J Med 2002;346(13):975–80.

52. Akl EA, Terrenato I, Barba M, et al. Extended perioperative thromboprophylaxis in patients with cancer. A systematic review. Thromb Haemost 2008;100(6): 1176–80.

53. Semrad TJ, O'Donnell R, Wun T, et al. Epidemiology of venous thromboembolism in 9489 patients with malignant glioma. J Neurosurg 2007;106(4):601–8.

54. Agnelli G, Piovella F, Buoncristiani P, et al. Enoxaparin plus compression stockings compared with compression stockings alone in the prevention of venous thromboembolism after elective neurosurgery. N Engl J Med 1998;339(2):80–5.

55. Clark-Pearson DL, DeLong E, Synan IS, et al. A controlled trial of two low-dose heparin regimens for the prevention of postoperative deep vein thrombosis. Obstet Gynecol 1990;75(4):684–9.

56. Clarke-Pearson DL, Coleman RE, Synan IS, et al. Venous thromboembolism prophylaxis in gynecologic oncology: a prospective, controlled trial of low-dose heparin. Am J Obstet Gynecol 1983;145(5):606–13.

57. Einstein MH, Pritts EA, Hartenbach EM. Venous thromboembolism prevention in gynecologic cancer surgery: a systematic review. Gynecol Oncol 2007;105(3): 813–9.

58. Hutten BA, Prins MH, Gent M, et al. Incidence of recurrent thromboembolic and bleeding complications among patients with venous thromboembolism in relation to both malignancy and achieved international normalized ratio: a retrospective analysis. J Clin Oncol 2000;18(17):3078–83.
59. Koopman MM, Prandoni P, Piovella F, et al. Treatment of venous thrombosis with intravenous unfractionated heparin administered in the hospital as compared with subcutaneous low-molecular-weight heparin administered at home. The Tasman Study Group. N Engl J Med 1996;334(11):682–7.
60. Gould MK, Dembitzer AD, Doyle RL, et al. Low-molecular-weight heparins compared with unfractionated heparin for treatment of acute deep venous thrombosis. A meta-analysis of randomized, controlled trials. Ann Intern Med 1999; 130(10):800–9.
61. Low-molecular-weight heparin in the treatment of patients with venous thromboembolism. The Columbus Investigators. N Engl J Med 1997;337(10):657–62.
62. Dolovich LR, Ginsberg JS, Douketis JD, et al. A meta-analysis comparing low-molecular-weight heparins with unfractionated heparin in the treatment of venous thromboembolism: examining some unanswered questions regarding location of treatment, product type, and dosing frequency. Arch Intern Med 2000;160(2): 181–8.
63. Merli G, Spiro TE, Olsson CG, et al. Subcutaneous enoxaparin once or twice daily compared with intravenous unfractionated heparin for treatment of venous thromboembolic disease. Ann Intern Med 2001;134(3):191–202.
64. Martel N, Lee J, Wells PS. Risk for heparin-induced thrombocytopenia with unfractionated and low-molecular-weight heparin thromboprophylaxis: a meta-analysis. Blood 2005;106(8):2710–5.
65. Akl EA, Barba M, Rohilla S, et al. Low-molecular-weight heparins are superior to vitamin K antagonists for the long term treatment of venous thromboembolism in patients with cancer: a Cochrane systematic review. J Exp Clin Cancer Res 2008; 27:21.
66. Lee AY, Levine MN, Baker RI, et al. Low-molecular-weight heparin versus a coumarin for the prevention of recurrent venous thromboembolism in patients with cancer. N Engl J Med 2003;349(2):146–53.
67. Louzada ML, Majeed H, Wells PS. Efficacy of low-molecular-weight heparin versus vitamin K antagonists for long term treatment of cancer-associated venous thromboembolism in adults: a systematic review of randomized controlled trials. Thromb Res 2009;123(6):837–44.
68. Wagman LD, Baird MF, Bennett CL, et al. Venous thromboembolic disease. NCCN. Clinical practice guidelines in oncology. J Natl Compr Canc Netw 2008; 6(8):716–53.
69. Kearon C, Kahn SR, Agnelli G, et al. Antithrombotic therapy for venous thromboembolic disease: American College of Chest Physicians evidence-based clinical practice guidelines (8th edition). Chest 2008;133(Suppl 6): 454S–545S.
70. Cronin CG, Lohan DG, Keane M, et al. Prevalence and significance of asymptomatic venous thromboembolic disease found on oncologic staging CT. AJR Am J Roentgenol 2007;189(1):162–70.
71. Douma RA, Kok MGM, Verberne LM, et al. Asymptomatic venous thromboembolism in cancer patients: prevalence and consequence. J Thromb Haemost 2009;7(Suppl 2) [abstract OC-MO-091]. Abstracts from the XXIIth International Society of Thrombosis and Haemostasis Congress; Boston. Available at: http://abstract.mci-group.

com/cgi-bin/mc/dq.pl?ccode=ISTH2009ABS&show=TKNAS. Accessed May 22, 2010.

72. Dentali F, Vitale J, Nitti C, et al. Prognostic relevance of asymptomatic VTE in cancer patients Journal of Thrombosis and Haemostasis. J Thromb Haemost 2009;7(Suppl 2). [abstract OC-MO-092]. Abstracts from the XXIIth International Society of Thrombosis and Haemostasis Congress; Boston. Available at: http://abstract.mci-group.com/cgi-bin/mc/dq.pl?ccode=ISTH2009ABS&show=TKNAS. Accessed May 22, 2010.

73. PREPIC Study Group. Eight-year follow-up of patients with permanent vena cava filters in the prevention of pulmonary embolism: the PREPIC (Prevention du Risque d'Embolie Pulmonaire par Interruption Cave) randomized study. Circulation. 2005;112(3):416–22.

74. De Cicco M, Matovic M, Balestreri L, et al. Central venous thrombosis: an early and frequent complication in cancer patients bearing long-term silastic catheter. A prospective study. Thromb Res 1997;86(2):101–13.

75. Luciani A, Clement O, Halimi P, et al. Catheter-related upper extremity deep venous thrombosis in cancer patients: a prospective study based on Doppler US. Radiology 2001;220(3):655–60.

76. Monreal M, Raventos A, Lerma R, et al. Pulmonary embolism in patients with upper extremity DVT associated to venous central lines—a prospective study. Thromb Haemost 1994;72(4):548–50.

77. Prandoni P, Bernardi E, Marchiori A, et al. The long term clinical course of acute deep vein thrombosis of the arm: prospective cohort study. BMJ 2004;329(7464): 484–5.

78. Bern MM, Lokich JJ, Wallach SR, et al. Very low doses of warfarin can prevent thrombosis in central venous catheters. A randomized prospective trial. Ann Intern Med 1990;112(6):423–8.

79. Monreal M, Alastrue A, Rull M, et al. Upper extremity deep venous thrombosis in cancer patients with venous access devices—prophylaxis with a low molecular weight heparin (Fragmin). Thromb Haemost 1996;75(2):251–3.

80. Verso M, Agnelli G, Bertoglio S, et al. Enoxaparin for the prevention of venous thromboembolism associated with central vein catheter: a double-blind, placebo-controlled, randomized study in cancer patients. J Clin Oncol 2005; 23(18):4057–62.

81. Karthaus M, Kretzschmar A, Kroning H, et al. Dalteparin for prevention of catheter-related complications in cancer patients with central venous catheters: final results of a double-blind, placebo-controlled phase III trial. Ann Oncol 2006;17(2):289–96.

82. Couban S, Goodyear M, Burnell M, et al. Randomized placebo-controlled study of low-dose warfarin for the prevention of central venous catheter-associated thrombosis in patients with cancer. J Clin Oncol 2005;23(18):4063–9.

83. Akl EA, Kamath G, Yosuico V, et al. Thromboprophylaxis for patients with cancer and central venous catheters: a systematic review and a meta-analysis. Cancer 2008;112(11):2483–92.

84. Carrier M, Tay J, Fergusson D, et al. Thromboprophylaxis for catheter-related thrombosis in patients with cancer: a systematic review of the randomized, controlled trials. J Thromb Haemost 2007;5(12):2552–4.

85. Chaukiyal P, Nautiyal A, Radhakrishnan S, et al. Thromboprophylaxis in cancer patients with central venous catheters. A systematic review and meta-analysis. Thromb Haemost 2008;99(1):38–43.

86. Savage KJ, Wells PS, Schulz V, et al. Outpatient use of low molecular weight heparin (dalteparin) for the treatment of deep vein thrombosis of the upper extremity. Thromb Haemost 1999;82(3):1008–10.

87. Debourdeau P, Farge-Bancel D, Bosquet L, et al. [2008 Standards, Options: recommendations for venous thromboembolic events (VTE) treatment and central venous catheter thrombosis (CVCT) management in cancer patients]. Bull Cancer 2008;95(7):750–61 [in French].

88. Kovacs MJ, Kahn SR, Rodger M, et al. A pilot study of central venous catheter survival in cancer patients using low-molecular-weight heparin (dalteparin) and warfarin without catheter removal for the treatment of upper extremity deep vein thrombosis (The Catheter Study). J Thromb Haemost 2007;5(8):1650–3.

Novel Risk Factors for Venous Thromboembolism

Alessandro Squizzato, MD, PhD*, Lorenza Brivio, MD,
Lorena Appio, MD, Francesco Dentali, MD

KEYWORDS

- Metabolic syndrome • JAK2 mutation • Hyperthyroidism
- Cushing syndrome • Venous thromboembolism • Risk factors

Venous thromboembolism (VTE), such as deep venous thrombosis (DVT) of the leg, pulmonary embolism (PE), and unusual-site thrombosis, is a common disorder.[1] Vein thrombus either arises spontaneously or is caused by well-known clinical conditions.[2] Orthopedic and cancer surgery, trauma and spinal cord injury, metastatic cancer, and acute medical illness are the most common settings in which thromboembolism occurs.[3] Besides major risk factors of VTE, several genetic and acquired minor risks have been identified.[2,3] Indeed, VTE is currently best understood as a multicausal disease in which more than one genetic or environmental condition coincides to produce clinically apparent thrombosis.[1] Therefore, weak thromboembolic risk factors may also be clinically relevant, especially if treatable. Novel risk factors for VTE, which were previously not described, are frequently reported. This article discusses the most promising risk factors for VTE: traditional cardiovascular risk factors, JAK2 mutation, and endocrine disorders (**Box 1**).

TRADITIONAL CARDIOVASCULAR RISK FACTORS

Arterial atherothrombotic disease and VTE were generally considered as separate entities from mechanistic and clinical points of view. However, several studies have recently challenged this dichotomy, suggesting a closer link between these 2 clinical conditions.[4–8]

Among traditional cardiovascular risk factors, only obesity and age have consistently been demonstrated to be independent risk factors for VTE.[9,10] In a prospective cohort study on 855 men, waist circumference greater than 100 cm was found to be associated with VTE (odds ratio [OR], 3.92; 95% confidence interval [CI], 2.10–7.29).[9]

The authors did not receive any financial support to write this manuscript.
Department of Clinical Medicine, Research Center on Thromboembolic Disorders and Antithrombotic Therapies, University of Insubria, UO Medicina I, Ospedale di Circolo, Viale Borri 57, Varese 21100, Italy
* Corresponding author. UO Medicina I, Ospedale di Circolo, Viale Borri 57, Varese 21100, Italy.
E-mail address: alexsquizzo@libero.it

Hematol Oncol Clin N Am 24 (2010) 709–716
doi:10.1016/j.hoc.2010.05.007
0889-8588/10/$ – see front matter © 2010 Elsevier Inc. All rights reserved.

hemonc.theclinics.com

Box 1
Novel persistent risk factors for VTE

Cardiovascular risk factors

- Hypertension
- Obesity
- Diabetes mellitus
- Dyslipidemia
- Smoking
- Metabolic syndrome

Ph− myeloproliferative disorders and JAK2V617F mutation

Endocrine disorders

- Thyroid dysfunction: hyperthyroidism and subclinical hypothyroidism
- Cushing syndrome
- Hyperprolactinemia

These results were confirmed by a similar study performed in 112,822 women in whom obesity was an independent predictor of PE[11] and by a population-based study in which obesity was strongly associated with the risk of DVT in men and women.[12]

Recently, several observational studies have also reported a positive association between dyslipidemia and VTE. Elevated levels of triglycerides and low levels of high-density lipoprotein (HDL) were found to increase the risk of VTE, whereas increased HDL levels may protect against VTE.[13–15] Doggen and colleagues[15] found that elevated serum triglyceride levels are associated with a doubling of the risk of VTE in postmenopausal women. Another study identified a link between increased levels of lipoprotein (a), a marker of atherosclerosis, and the risk of unprovoked VTE (OR, 2.1; 95% CI, 1.4–3.2).[16] Observational studies have also reported a positive association between DVT and/or PE and diabetes,[17] arterial hypertension, and smoking.

However, other studies have failed to find a significant association between these traditional cardiovascular risk factors and VTE. For example, in a study on 19,293 subjects, a higher incidence of VTE was associated with obesity (OR, 2.27; 95% CI, 1.57–3.28) and diabetes (OR, 1.7; 95% CI, 1.2–2.4) but not with hypertension at 8 years of follow-up,[18] and in another study that enrolled 18,662 male physicians, VTE was associated with obesity but not with hypertension, hypercholesterolemia, diabetes, or smoking at 20 years of follow-up.[19]

To further assess the strength of the evidence supporting the association between cardiovascular risk factors and VTE, Ageno and colleagues[20] recently performed a systematic review and a meta-analysis of the literature. The prevalence of 5 major established risk factors for atherosclerosis (obesity, arterial hypertension, diabetes mellitus, smoking, and dyslipidemia) was compared in patients with VTE and in controls based on data from 21 selected case-control and cohort studies, including a total of more than 60,000 patients and controls. Obesity (OR, 2.33; 95% CI, 1.68–3.24), hypertension (OR, 1.51; 95% CI, 1.23–1.85), and diabetes mellitus (OR, 1.42; 95% CI, 1.12–1.77) were associated with VTE. There was no significant association with smoking (OR, 1.18; 95% CI, 0.95–1.46). Hypercholesterolemia was not associated with an increased risk of VTE (OR, 1.16; 95% CI, 0.67–2.02), but the weighted mean in HDL cholesterol levels was significantly lower in patients with VTE than in controls (−2.86 mg/dL; 95% CI, −4.34 to −1.38, $P<.05$). Likewise, triglyceride levels were, on an average, 21.0 mg/dL (95% CI, 10.0–31.0) higher in patients with VTE than in controls. No significant difference was observed for low-density lipoprotein cholesterol levels in both the groups, although the small number of included studies did not allow any meaningful conclusion.

Although these results should be considered with caution because of the design of included studies and because of the significant heterogeneity among the studies for all variables apart from diabetes, there is reasonable biologic plausibility underlying the hypothesis that VTE is associated with risk factors for cardiovascular disease. Obesity and diabetes are known to predispose patients to hypercoagulable and inflammatory states, hypertension may induce endothelial dysfunction, and dyslipidemia is also associated with hypercoagulability and endothelial dysfunction. All such effects, in particular when combined, may induce a prothrombotic effect that could also predispose patients to an increased risk of VTE. This association might help explain, in part, the pathogenesis of many idiopathic episodes of VTE.

Recent studies have addressed the relationship between VTE and the metabolic syndrome, which is a cluster of cardiovascular risk factors, including obesity, hyperlipidemia, hypertension, and hyperglycemia. Ageno and colleagues[21] observed a significantly higher prevalence of this syndrome among patients with idiopathic DVT than among matched controls without venous thrombosis. These findings were confirmed by the results of 2 other case-control studies in European and Korean patients.[22,23]

Although recent trials[24] have suggested that drugs traditionally used for primary and secondary prevention of atherosclerotic disease (such as statins) may also reduce the incidence of VTE, further studies are warranted to confirm these preliminary findings.

PHILADELPHIA-NEGATIVE MYELOPROLIFERATIVE NEOPLASMS AND *JAK2* MUTATION

Splanchnic vein thromboses (SVTs), which include portal vein thrombosis, mesenteric vein thrombosis, and thrombosis of the hepatic veins (causing Budd-Chiari syndrome), are frequently the first manifestations of Philadelphia-negative (Ph−) myeloproliferative neoplasms (MPNs), polycythemia vera (PV), and essential thrombocythemia (ET).[25] Overall, Ph− MPNs are among the most common causes of Budd-Chiari syndrome and portal vein thrombosis, being found in up to 50% and 25% of the patients, respectively.[26] The identification of occult MPNs in patients with VTE has traditionally been based on bone marrow biopsy findings and endogenous erythroid colony formation assessment.[27] The discovery of the gain-of-function *JAK2V617F* mutation, found in approximately 90% of patients with PV and in 50% of those with ET or primary myelofibrosis (PM), has modified the diagnostic approach to Ph− MPNs.[28]

Several studies and a recent meta-analysis have explored whether screening for the *JAK2V617F* mutation in patients presenting with venous thrombosis without overt MPN is justified.[29] The mean prevalence of the *JAK2* mutation was 32.7% (95% CI, 25.5%–35.9%) in patients with SVT; the mutation was associated with an increased risk of SVT (OR, 53.98; 95% CI, 13.10–222.45) and with a subsequent diagnosis of MPNs in many of these patients. The *JAK2* mutation was rare in patients with VTE in other locations (frequency, 0.88% to 2.57%).[29] These results suggest that screening for the *JAK2* mutation be considered in patients with SVT because this mutation is a strong predictor of a subsequent development of an MPN. A recent meta-analysis comparing patients with and without the mutation explored the mutation's possible role as a procoagulant in ET and in PM.[30] In patients with ET, *JAK2V617F* mutation was associated with a significant increased risk of thrombosis (OR, 1.92; 95% CI, 1.45–2.53), both of venous (OR, 2.49; 95% CI, 1.71–3.61) and arterial (OR, 1.77; 95% CI, 1.29–2.43) vessels. In patients with PM, the presence of *JAK2V617F* mutation was associated with a trend toward increased risk of thrombosis (OR, 1.76; 95% CI, 0.91–3.41).[30] The recommendation for screening is strengthened by the observation that the concomitant presence of portal hypertension and hypersplenism could mask the increase in blood cell counts, which is the cardinal manifestation of the MPNs.[31]

Why the *JAK2* mutation is associated with SVT is unknown. The mutation causes constitutive activation of *JAK2*, which in turn results in cytokine-independent myelo-proliferation, mobilization of blood cell progenitors, and spontaneous formation of endogenous erythroid colonies leading to the development of the MPN.[32] How these factors predict for splanchnic but not other forms of VTE is unknown.

ENDOCRINE DYSFUNCTIONS

Endocrine disorders can influence the hemostatic balance. Several abnormal coagulation test results and clinical events have been observed in patients with abnormal hormone levels.[33] The best evidence is available for hyperthyroidism and endogenous Cushing syndrome.[34,35] An imbalance in coagulation and fibrinolysis has been shown in hyperprolactinemia, growth hormone excess or deficiency, exogenous hypercortisolism, pheochromocytoma, primary hyperaldosteronism, and hyperparathyroidism.[36,37]

Thyroid Dysfunction

The link between the hemostatic system and thyroid diseases has been known since the beginning of the last century. The first clinical association was described in 1913, when Kaliebe reported an episode of cerebral vein thrombosis in a thyrotoxic patient.[38] Several elements of the process of thrombus formation may be involved.[39] Thyroid dysfunction and autoimmunity may modify physiologic processes of hemostasis and lead to thrombosis. Secondary antiphospholipid syndrome has been associated with autoimmune thyroid disorders, but the main influence of thyroid hormone on the coagulation-fibrinolytic system is mediated by the interaction between the hormone and its receptors.[40] A recent review systematically summarized published studies on this topic, both for hyperthyroidism and hypothyroidism.[34] A total of 39 case-control studies and 24 interventional cohort studies, none of high quality, were analyzed. A total of 19 tests were investigated in the medium-quality studies. Overall, these tests revealed a tendency to a hypercoagulable state for overt hyperthyroidism, and conversely, a hypocoagulable state for overt hypothyroidism.[34]

Additional information about the influence of thyroid hormones on coagulation comes from 2 interventional studies performed in healthy volunteers.[41,42] Although only a few tests were performed and thyroid hormones were administered for a relatively short period of 2 weeks, a clear increase of factor VIII level, von Willebrand antigen level and activity, and tissue plasminogen activator (tPA) antigen level was observed.

In a pilot cross-sectional study, Squizzato and colleagues[43] assessed the frequency of overt and subclinical thyroid dysfunction in 50 consecutive patients with a previous unprovoked DVT, 50 patients with a previous DVT secondary to other risk factors, and 50 subjects in whom DVT was ruled out. In each patient, thyroid hormones and thyroid autoantibodies were assayed. Previously unrecognized subclinical hypothyroidism was diagnosed in 7 patients (14.0%) with unprovoked DVT, in 1 patient (2%) with

DVT secondary to other risk factors, and in 1 (2%) patient of the control group (OR for subclinical hypothyroidism at multivariate analysis between unprovoked DVT and controls, 5.54; 95% CI, 0.6–52.6). Unfortunately, no conclusion could be drawn for hyperthyroidism because of the limited sample size. Taken together, published data are insufficient to recommend routine assessment of thyroid function in patients with thromboembolic disorders.

Endogenous Hypercortisolism

Cushing syndrome, which is characterized by lengthy and inappropriate exposure to excessive concentrations of free glucocorticoids, is an uncommon disease with an estimated incidence ranging from 0.7 to 2.4 cases per million per year, depending on the population studied.[44] This low incidence makes alterations in the coagulation and fibrinolytic system in patients with Cushing syndrome extremely difficult to investigate, and even more so for clinical outcomes of venous or arterial thrombosis.

In a recent systematic review, the authors found high levels of factor VIII, factor IX, and von Willebrand factor, with subsequent shortening of activated partial thromboplastin time and evidence of enhanced thrombin generation in patients with Cushing syndrome.[35] Levels tended to normalize after successful treatment. Small increases in plasminogen activity, tPA antigen level, α2-antiplasmin activity, and plasminogen activator inhibitor (PAI) 1 activity were observed during glucocorticoid excess, but the net effect on fibrinolytic activity remained uncertain.[35] Erem and colleagues[45] aimed to further elucidate ways in which endogenous glucocorticoid excess may affect fibrinolysis. In this study, the investigators failed to show any significant change in thrombin-activated fibrinolytic inhibitor levels in 24 patients with Cushing syndrome and in 24 healthy sex- and age-matched controls. However, these investigators confirm earlier observations of a glucocorticoid-induced increase in PAI-1 levels, which are positively correlated with midnight serum cortisol concentration in the patients with Cushing syndrome. This observation was further supported by a recent study by Kastelan and colleagues[46] on 33 patients with Cushing syndrome and 31 healthy controls. Besides a significant increase in PAI-1 levels, the investigators found high levels of prothrombin and factors V, VIII, IX, XI, and XII in patients with Cushing syndrome.

Cushing syndrome is associated with a 4-fold increase in the risk of death (standardized mortality ratio, 3.8; 95% CI, 2.5–17.9), with cardiovascular disease being the most frequent cause of death.[47,48] Although this fact is best explained by the accelerated atherosclerosis associated with glucocorticoid excess, glucocorticoid-induced alterations in hemostasis may also contribute to the increased risk. Endogenous glucocorticoid excess has also been associated with an increased risk of venous thrombosis, further increasing the risk of cardiovascular morbidity. Reported risk rate of postoperative VTE in patients with Cushing syndrome undergoing transsphenoidal surgery or laparoscopic adrenal procedures seems to be slightly higher than the rate of symptomatic VTE found in patients undergoing similar surgical procedure for other endocrine disorders. In fact, the risk rate of VTE in patients with Cushing syndrome is comparable to the rate after major orthopedic surgery (1.3%–4.4% after total hip or knee replacement despite thromboprophylaxis), which is considered a procedure at high risk of VTE.[49] Whether this observation justifies extended duration or more intense thromboprophylaxis in patients with Cushing syndrome remains to be elucidated. Until definitive recommendations on thromboprophylaxis in Cushing syndrome are provided, an adequate thromboembolic risk assessment should be performed for each patient at the time of diagnosis to decide on the best prophylactic strategy.

SUMMARY

VTE can be considered as a multicausal disease involving various inherited and acquired prothrombotic conditions.[1] Although greater emphasis has classically been given to traditional thrombophilic risk factors, there is increasing recognition of less typical precipitating conditions and events.[50] In this article, the authors focus on the most promising, persistent, and potentially treatable novel risk factors.

Observational studies have suggested that several traditional cardiovascular risk factors, including obesity, diabetes, hypertension, dyslipidemia, and smoking, may be independent risk factors for VTE also. However, evidence is conflicting, and larger prospective studies are warranted to confirm or refute these associations.

JAK2 mutation is uncommon in patients with DVT, PE, or cerebral vein thrombosis, and screening for the mutation in these patients does not seem justified. The JAK2 mutation is frequent in patients with SVT, and because it is a strong predictor of a subsequent diagnosis of an MPN, patients with SVT should be screened for this mutation.

Among endocrine dysfunctions, only hyperthyroidism and endogenous hypercortisolism seem to be associated with an increased risk of VTE. Published data are, however, insufficient to recommend routine checking of endocrine status in patients with thromboembolic disorders.

Further evidence is warranted to conclusively define the true contribution of all such conditions to the cause of acute episodes of VTE and to provide practical recommendation for its primary and secondary prevention in patients with these novel risk factors; however, it seems reasonable to conclude that the concomitant presence of such conditions with one or more additional risk factors for VTE might be clinically relevant.

REFERENCES

1. Rosendaal FR. Venous thrombosis: a multicausal disease. Lancet 1999;353: 1167–73.
2. Kyrle PA, Eichinger S. Deep vein thrombosis. Lancet 2005;365(9465):1163–74.
3. Tapson VF. Acute pulmonary embolism. N Engl J Med 2008;358(10):1037–52.
4. Prandoni P. Links between arterial and venous disease. J Intern Med 2007;262: 341–50.
5. Jeries-Sanchez C. Venous and arterial thrombosis: a continuous spectrum of the same disease? Eur Heart J 2005;26:3–4.
6. Agnelli G, Becattini C. Venous thromboembolism and atherosclerosis: common denominators or different diseases? J Thromb Haemost 2006;4:1886–90.
7. Lowe GD. Arterial disease and venous thrombosis: are they related, and if so, what should we do about it? J Thromb Haemost 2006;4:1882–5.
8. Prandoni P. Venous thromboembolism and atherosclerosis: is there a link? J Thromb Haemost 2007;5(Suppl 1):270–5.
9. Hansson PO, Eriksson H, Welin L, et al. Smoking and abdominal obesity: risk factors for venous thromboembolism among middle-aged men: "the Study of Men Born in 1913". Arch Intern Med 1999;159:1886–90.
10. Samama MM. An epidemiologic study of risk factors for deep vein thrombosis in medical outpatients: the Sirius study. Arch Intern Med 2000;160:3415–20.
11. Goldhaber SZ, Grodstein F, Stampfer MJ, et al. A prospective study of risk factors for pulmonary embolism in women. JAMA 1997;277:642–5.
12. Stein PD, Beemath A, Olson RE. Obesity as a risk factor in venous thromboembolism. Am J Med 2005;118:978–80.

13. Vaya A, Mira Y, Ferrando F, et al. Hyperlipidemia and venous thromboembolism in patients lacking thrombophilic risk factors. Br J Haematol 2002;118:255–9.
14. Deguchi H, Pecheniuk NM, Elias DJ, et al. High-density lipoprotein deficiency and dyslipoproteinemia associated with venous thrombosis in men. Circulation 2005;112:893–9.
15. Doggen CJ, Smith NL, Lemaitre RN, et al. Serum lipid levels and the risk of venous thrombosis. Arterioscler Thromb Vasc Biol 2004;24:1970–5.
16. Marcucci R, Liotta AA, Cellai AP, et al. Increased plasma levels of lipoprotein(a) and the risk of idiopathic and recurrent venous thromboembolism. Am J Med 2003;115:601–5.
17. Petrauskiene V, Falk M, Waernbaum I, et al. The risk of venous thromboembolism is markedly elevated in patients with diabetes. Diabetologia 2005;48:1017–21.
18. Tsai AW, Cushman M, Rosamond WD, et al. Cardiovascular risk factors and venous thromboembolism incidence. Arch Intern Med 2002;162:1182–9.
19. Glynn RJ, Rosner B. Comparison of risk factors for the competing risks of coronary heart disease, stroke, and venous thromboembolism. Am J Epidemiol 2005;162:975–82.
20. Ageno W, Becattini C, Brighton T, et al. Cardiovascular risk factors and venous thromboembolism: a meta-analysis. Circulation 2008;117:93–102.
21. Ageno W, Prandoni P, Romualdi E, et al. The metabolic syndrome and the risk of venous thrombosis: a case-control study. J Thromb Haemost 2006;4:1914–8.
22. Ay C, Tengler T, Vormittag R, et al. Venous thromboembolism—a manifestation of the metabolic syndrome. Haematologica 2007;92:374–80.
23. Jang MJ, Choi WI, Bang SM, et al. Metabolic syndrome is associated with venous thromboembolism in the Korean population. Arterioscler Thromb Vasc Biol 2009;29(3):311–5.
24. Squizzato A, Galli M, Romualdi E, et al. Statins, fibrates, and venous thromboembolism: a meta-analysis. Eur Heart J 2010;31(10):1248–56.
25. Polycythemia vera: the natural history of 1213 patients followed for 20 years. Gruppo Italiano Studio Policitemia. Ann Intern Med 1995;123:656–64.
26. Valla D, Casadevall N, Huisse MG, et al. Etiology of portal vein thrombosis in adults: a prospective evaluation of primary myeloproliferative disorders. Gastroenterology 1988;94:1063–9.
27. Chait Y, Condat B, Cazals-Hatem D, et al. Relevance of the criteria commonly used to diagnose myeloproliferative disorder in patients with splanchnic vein thrombosis. Br J Haematol 2005;129:553–60.
28. James C, Ugo V, Le Couedic JP, et al. A unique clonal JAK2 mutation leading to constitutive signalling causes polycythaemia vera. Nature 2005;434:1144–8.
29. Dentali F, Squizzato A, Brivio L, et al. JAK2V617F mutation for the early diagnosis of Ph- myeloproliferative neoplasms in patients with venous thromboembolism: a meta-analysis. Blood 2009;113(22):5617–23.
30. Lussana F, Caberlon S, Pagani C, et al. Association of V617F Jak2 mutation with the risk of thrombosis among patients with essential thrombocythaemia or idiopathic myelofibrosis: a systematic review. Thromb Res 2009;124(4):409–17.
31. Hexner EO. JAK2 V617F: implications for thrombosis in myeloproliferative diseases. Curr Opin Hematol 2007;14:450–4.
32. Austin SK, Lambert JR. The JAK2(V617F) mutation and thrombosis. Br J Haematol 2008;143:307–20.
33. Squizzato A, Gerdes VE, Ageno W, et al. The coagulation system in endocrine disorders: a narrative review. Intern Emerg Med 2007;2:76–83.

34. Squizzato A, Romualdi E, Büller HR, et al. Clinical review: thyroid dysfunction and effects on coagulation and fibrinolysis: a systematic review. Clin Endocrinol Metab 2007;92(7):2415–20.

35. Van Zaane B, Nur E, Squizzato A, et al. Hypercoagulable state in Cushing's syndrome: a systematic review. J Clin Endocrinol Metab 2009;94:2743–50.

36. Targher G, Pichiri I, Zoppini G, et al. Hemostatic and fibrinolytic abnormalities in endocrine diseases: a narrative review. Semin Thromb Hemost 2009;35:605–12.

37. van Zaane B, Reuwer AQ, Büller HR, et al. Hormones and cardiovascular disease: a shift in paradigm with clinical consequences? Semin Thromb Hemost 2009;35:478–87.

38. Squizzato A, Gerdes VEA, Brandjes DPM, et al. Thyroid diseases and cerebrovascular disease. Stroke 2005;36:2302–10.

39. Hofbauer LC, Heufelder AE. Coagulation disorders in thyroid diseases. Eur J Endocrinol 1997;136:1–7.

40. Shih CH, Chen SL, Yen CC, et al. Thyroid hormone receptor dependent transcriptional regulation of fibrinogen and coagulation proteins. Endocrinology 2004;145: 2804–14.

41. Rogers JS II, Stanley RS. Factor VIII activity in normal volunteers receiving oral thyroid hormone. J Lab Clin Med 1983;102:444–9.

42. Graninger W, Pirich KR, Speiser W. Effect of thyroid hormones on plasma protein concentrations in man. J Clin Endocrinol Metab 1986;63:407–11.

43. Squizzato A, Romualdi E, Piantanida E, et al. Subclinical hypothyroidism and deep venous thrombosis. A pilot cross-sectional study. Thromb Haemost 2007; 97(5):803–6.

44. Newell-Price J, Bertagna X, Grossman AB, et al. Cushing's syndrome. Lancet 2006;367(9522):1605–17.

45. Erem C, Nuhoglu I, Yilmaz M, et al. Blood coagulation and fibrinolysis in patients with Cushing's syndrome: increased plasminogen activator inhibitor-1, decreased tissue factor pathway inhibitor, and unchanged thrombin-activatable fibrinolysis inhibitor levels. J Endocrinol Invest 2009;32:169–74.

46. Kastelan D, Dusek T, Kraljevic I, et al. Hypercoagulability in Cushing's syndrome: the role of specific haemostatic and fibrinolytic markers. Endocrine 2009;36:70–4.

47. Dekkers OM, Biermasz NR, Pereira AM, et al. Mortality in patients treated for Cushing's disease is increased, compared with patients treated for nonfunctioning pituitary macroadenoma. J Clin Endocrinol Metab 2007;92:976–81.

48. Etxabe J, Vazquez JA. Morbidity and mortality in Cushing's disease: an epidemiological approach. Clin Endocrinol (Oxf) 1994;40:479–84.

49. Geerts WH, Bergqvist D, Pineo GF, et al. Prevention of venous thromboembolism: American College of Chest Physicians Evidence-Based Clinical Practice Guidelines (8th Edition). Chest 2008;133(Suppl 6):381S–453S.

50. Lippi G, Franchini M, Favaloro EJ. Unsuspected triggers of venous thromboembolism–trivial or not so trivial? Semin Thromb Hemost 2009;35(7):597–604.

Optimizing Use of Current Anticoagulants

Daniel M. Witt, PharmD, FCCP, BCPS, CACP

KEYWORDS

- Warfarin • Administration and dosage • Adverse effects
- Anticoagulants • Drug effects • Drug therapy • Therapeutic use

For decades, vitamin K antagonists (VKAs) like warfarin sodium have served well as the oral anticoagulant drugs of choice for prevention and treatment of thromboembolic disease.[1] Despite excellent clinical efficacy, warfarin remains a difficult treatment to deliver. Because of wide intra- and interindividual variability and the small differential separating beneficial and toxic therapeutic effects, warfarin is classified as a narrow therapeutic index drug. Consequently, frequent assessment of the effect of warfarin on the coagulation system, as measured clinically by the international normalized ratio (INR), is required for the duration of treatment.[1] Frequent INR monitoring and follow-up have potential negative effects on quality of life. The pharmacokinetics and pharmacodynamics of warfarin are altered by several factors, including diet, alcohol use, many medications, and concurrent illnesses.[1] Because of these challenges and fear of bleeding complications, warfarin remains underused despite an increasing number of patients who might benefit from its use.[2] The many liabilities associated with warfarin therapy have fueled ongoing efforts to develop effective oral anticoagulants that are clinically easier to use.[3]

New oral anticoagulants (eg, dabigatran and rivaroxaban) have been introduced for selected indications, namely orthopedic thromboprophylaxis, in Canada and Europe and are in different phases of testing for other indications and in preparation for introduction in the United States. There is speculation that the introduction of newer, easier-to-use anticoagulants will eliminate the need for warfarin.[4] Although the cost of newer agents is yet to be defined in the US market, they will be more expensive than warfarin, which is available as a generic drug. Results of clinical trials comparing new anticoagulants with adjusted-dose warfarin therapy have largely reported similar efficacy and safety,[5,6] particularly when warfarin therapy is well managed. Patients with stable INR control have been shown to experience significantly fewer anticoagulation therapy-related complications compared with patients with less stable INR

Clinical Pharmacy Services & Research, Department of Pharmacy, Kaiser Permanente Colorado, 16601 East Centretech Parkway, Aurora, CO 80011, USA
E-mail address: dan.m.witt@kp.org

Hematol Oncol Clin N Am 24 (2010) 717–726
doi:10.1016/j.hoc.2010.05.010
0889-8588/10/$ – see front matter © 2010 Elsevier Inc. All rights reserved.

control.[7,8] Data from retrospective studies further support the use of INR stability to accurately predict reductions in adverse events.[9] Therefore, before a tried-and-true therapeutic modality like warfarin with decades of accumulated clinical experience is abandoned in favor of novel newer agents, measures to ensure optimal use of warfarin should be fully explored. In addition, warfarin remains the therapy of choice for patients with mechanical heart valves and for those who experience therapeutic failure on the newer agents. This article examines various approaches to optimize the clinical use of warfarin.

INITIATION OF THERAPY

Selecting appropriate candidates for warfarin therapy is an important first step in achieving optimal anticoagulation. A valid indication for anticoagulation therapy should exist. Although the preceding statement should be intuitive, patients receiving atrial fibrillation with low underlying stroke risk likely receive minimal net benefit from warfarin therapy.[10] Therefore, before initiating therapy, careful weighing of the risk and benefits of warfarin therapy is required.

Before initiating therapy a thorough patient assessment should be performed, including a comprehensive medical, family, medication history (including dietary supplements and over-the-counter drugs); social, lifestyle, and employment profile; and health beliefs and attitudes, level of understanding, health literacy, personal health motivation, and health care resources.[11] The risks of warfarin therapy may outweigh benefits in patients with a previous history of medication nonadherence, bleeding risk factors, history of falls, significant alcohol consumption, memory impairment, and lack of adequate support from family members or caregivers. Validated tools exist for conducting formal bleeding risk assessment.[12,13] Patients and/or their caregivers should be involved in the discussion of the risks and benefits associated with warfarin therapy and should agree with the decision to initiate therapy.[11] Some anticoagulation providers require new patients to sign a contract indicating their commitment to adhere to the requirements of warfarin therapy.

PATIENT EDUCATION

When patients are actively involved in, understand, and take responsibility for their care the likelihood of INR stability is improved.[14] Patient education is an essential component in quality management of the anticoagulated patient. Because it is time consuming for clinicians and overwhelming for patients, educating the anticoagulated patient is often neglected.[15] A formalized warfarin education curriculum based on established models may be more likely to improve patient's knowledge level compared with an ad hoc approach.[16] Specific warfarin knowledge-assessment tools have been developed to help assess patients' educational needs.[17] Efforts to educate patients regarding warfarin therapy should continue throughout treatment.

INDUCTION OF THERAPY

Various algorithms aimed at quickly achieving therapeutic INR values during warfarin therapy induction have been developed.[18–21] The size of the initial warfarin dose is a key differentiation between the various available algorithms. Regardless of the size of the initial warfarin dose, a key component of successful warfarin initiation is a structured initiation process that incorporates frequent INR assessments (at least 2–3 times per week) with subsequent warfarin dose titration.[1]

Genetic variability among patients, specifically variants of cytochrome P450 2C9 (CYP2C9) and vitamin K epoxide reductase (VKORC1), plays a role in determining the eventual required therapeutic warfarin dose.[22] Determining CYP2C9 and VKORC1 status before initiating warfarin therapy has been enthusiastically promoted as a means to improve the accuracy of initial warfarin dose selection.[22,23] However, the promise of genotype-guided initial warfarin dosing remains largely unfulfilled and current evidence does not support its routine use.[24]

MAINTENANCE OF THERAPY

Standardization of follow-up procedures using checklists, flow diagrams, or computerized tracking systems should be used to ensure consistency of warfarin management.[25] Before determining warfarin dose instructions, a thorough assessment of the various factors that influence warfarin dosing requirements (eg, diet, concurrent illness, other medications, alcohol use, and adherence to dosing instructions) should be completed, especially for out-of-range INRs.[11] Patients should also be assessed regularly for signs and symptoms of bleeding or clotting complications.

Maintenance Dosing Algorithms

Validated algorithms for adjusting warfarin doses should be incorporated into operating procedures.[25,26] Using algorithms reduces clinician variation in the management of warfarin doses and can improve the stability of INR control. Frequent warfarin dose changes in response to slightly out-of-range INRs (eg, 1.8–1.9 or 3.1–3.2 for target INR range of 2.0–3.0) perturbs INR control, setting up a cycle of dose adjustment and readjustment.[27,28] It has been suggested that for target INR range of 2.0 to 3.0, an optimal maintenance dose management strategy would be to change warfarin doses only when the INR is 1.7 or less or 3.3 or greater.[27,28] It has been further suggested that INR reductions greater than 20% be avoided in most circumstances.[28] Target INR ranges should be evidence based (eg, 2.0–3.0 and 2.5–3.5 in most cases).[1]

It is common practice to instruct patients with otherwise stable INR control who present with a slightly out-of-range INR to skip or boost the dose of warfarin one time before reverting back to the usual dosing schedule.[29] Although this behavior may bring the INR more rapidly back into the therapeutic range, a recent study showed the net effect on the next measured INR was unimportant compared with simply continuing the usual warfarin dose alone.[29] Furthermore, the clinical benefit of this practice is probably negligible because of the low risk of bleeding or thromboembolic complications associated with short periods outside the therapeutic range.[30,31]

Studies of computer-assisted warfarin dosing have consistently shown improvements in INR control compared with manual dosing.[32–37] When possible, computer-assisted or paper-based algorithms are preferred to an ad hoc dosing approach.[25] Evidence-based guidelines should be used to establish a systematic approach to responding to extreme INR values (eg, >5.0 and <1.5).[1]

INR Recall Interval

Likewise, a systematic approach should be used to determine the interval between INR tests that maximizes the amount of time patients spend within their therapeutic range. The 4-week maximum recall interval between INR measurements recommended by consensus guidelines is not evidence based, having evolved instead from routine clinical practice and expert opinion.[1,38,39] The weekly INR testing that has been suggested for patients who self-monitor INRs using portable fingerstick INR monitors is probably unnecessary for patients showing long-term INR stability.[27,40]

High-frequency INR testing raises the likelihood of measuring slightly out-of-range INR values (which as discussed previously can lead to unnecessary warfarin dose changes) and unnecessarily increases the costs associated with warfarin therapy. Evidence supports less frequent INR monitoring for patients with stable INR control.[7,8,27,41,42] Recent studies have shown that a stable subgroup of patients treated with warfarin can be identified, in whom allowing 8-week INR recall intervals would be reasonable.[7,8] Stable INR control in these studies was associated with age greater than 70 years, target INRs less than 3.0, and lower chronic disease burden. In the United Kingdom INR recall intervals of up to 90 days are routinely used in patients with stable INR control.[43] Therefore, INR recall intervals should be individually tailored based on proven INR control rather than being fixed at some arbitrary minimum frequency, such as 4 weeks.[42]

Drug and Dietary Interactions

Warfarin therapy is complicated by administration of drugs that interfere with its pharmacokinetic and pharmacodynamic properties, leading to loss of INR control.[1] Avoidance of interacting drug therapy is preferred, but not always feasible.[44] Although there is no clinical standard for managing warfarin therapy when interacting drugs are coadministered, 2 strategies are generally used.[1,45] The conventional approach involves increasing INR monitoring frequency with reactive warfarin dose adjustment based on INR response.[44] Alternatively, the warfarin dose can be preemptively increased or decreased on initiation of the interacting medication in addition to increasing the frequency of INR monitoring in anticipation of subsequent INR increase or decrease.[46] When drugs with a known strong tendency to affect the INR, such as cotrimoxazole, are coadministered, preemptive warfarin dose alteration may reduce the likelihood of subsequent nontherapeutic INRs.[46] Conversely, using timely INR monitoring to identify patients with altered INR response then reactively adjusting the warfarin dose may be preferred for interacting medications with less predictable effects on the INR, such as levofloxacin.[46] The value of the first follow-up INR following initiation of an interacting drug may be less important than longitudinal INR control during the weeks that follow. Evidence indicates that the risk of major bleeding in patients with INRs between 4.5 and 10.0 and the risk of thromboembolism associated with isolated subtherapeutic INRs are low provided steps are taken to rapidly restore therapeutic anticoagulation.[30,31] Therefore, ensuring timely INR monitoring and adjusting doses of warfarin when necessary is of primary importance. Application of pharmacokinetic and pharmacodynamic principles is necessary to determine how long increased INR monitoring frequency is required. For interacting drugs like rifampin and amiodarone, prolonged effects on the INR response of warfarin are possible, necessitating careful INR monitoring for weeks or months.[47,48]

Some warfarin drug interactions do not alter the INR response but rather increase the risk for bleeding complications; this is perhaps best illustrated by concomitant administration of warfarin and aspirin therapy. Many patients receiving warfarin therapy also have indications for antiplatelet therapy, for example coronary artery and cerebrovascular disease, and some patients take a daily aspirin without knowledge of their anticoagulant provider. One study showed that concurrent administration of antiplatelet therapy was present in nearly 40% of patients receiving warfarin enrolled in an anticoagulation monitoring service.[49] In most cases, adding aspirin to warfarin therapy merely increases the risk of significant bleeding without further reducing thromboembolic risk.[50] Clinicians should carefully consider whether adding antiplatelet therapy to warfarin therapy is warranted and should clearly document aspirin use or nonuse in all patients prescribed warfarin.

Dietary vitamin K intake can affect the INR response to warfarin.[44] This drug-food interaction can be clinically relevant and independently interfere with INR stability.[51,52] The precise amount of dietary vitamin K that should be ingested by patients receiving warfarin has not been definitively established and this component of achieving optimal INR stability is frequently overlooked.[51] A recent study reported that a dietary vitamin K-guided strategy for adjusting oral anticoagulation therapy, in lieu of the conventional approach of altering oral anticoagulant doses, was feasible, safe, and may result in increased INR control.[51] The strategy involved an assessment of vitamin K intake using a validated instrument that evaluated usual consumption of 16 vitamin K-rich foods. Based on this assessment, patients with low or high INR values were instructed to half or double the consumption frequency of vitamin K-rich foods. Oral anticoagulant dose remained unaltered. Patients randomized to the vitamin K-guided strategy had the same magnitude and direction of INR variation as patients randomized to the conventional anticoagulant medication dose adjustment arm. A higher proportion of patients in the vitamin K-guided strategy group reached a prespecified INR target at study conclusion compared with conventional management (74%, vs 58%, respectively, $P = .04$). A separate approach involving daily administration of vitamin K supplements (100 to 200 µg/d) has also been shown to improve INR control for patients with unexplained variability in response to warfarin.[1,53] Daily vitamin K supplementation in this manner is believed to override any variability in dietary vitamin K intake, allowing eventual stabilization of the INR response following a period of careful monitoring and warfarin dose titration.[53] In determining whether a patient with variable INR control is a candidate for daily supplemental vitamin K, known causes of INR variability (eg, poor adherence to warfarin therapy, drug interactions, changes in health status, and alcohol abuse), should be first excluded. Although more study is required to clarify the role of vitamin K-based strategies for improving INR control, for patients with persistently unstable INR control, efforts targeting vitamin K intake may yield improvement.[51,53]

COORDINATION OF CARE

Managing warfarin therapy is a complex enterprise. Policies and procedures are necessary to reduce variability and potential lapses in the delivery of care.[11] Policies and procedures should be reviewed and revised regularly. Coordination of anticoagulation therapy requires seamless communication between all involved health care system members and patients and their caregivers.[11] Communication failures can result in poor patient outcomes. A structured, efficient system for scheduling and tracking anticoagulated patients should be used to minimize the possibility that a patient could be lost to follow-up, even for a brief period.[11]

Most patients receiving warfarin therapy are managed by their own physician, along with all other patients in the practice and with no organized program of management, education, or follow-up.[54] The results of many studies have reported better outcomes in patients when anticoagulant therapy is managed by a specialized anticoagulation management service (AMS) than by the usual care provided by the prescribing physician.[55] An AMS is typically staffed by pharmacists, nurses, midlevel providers, or advanced practice nurses. This model allows a core of individuals with specialized training to regularly interact with, evaluate, and educate patients taking warfarin. In addition, meticulous tracking allows observation and identification of individual and population trends in dose-response, medication interactions, adverse events, and so forth.[4] Even when AMS care is unavailable, health care providers who manage warfarin therapy should strive to model the systematic and coordinated care provided

Table 1	
Anticoagulation therapy consensus guidelines and recommendations	
References	**Comment**
American College of Chest Physicians Consensus Conference on Antithrombotic Therapy[1]	Comprehensive guideline updated regularly that is widely regarded as the definitive resource for graded recommendations pertaining to anticoagulation therapy
Consensus Guidelines for the Delivery of Optimized Anticoagulant Therapy[11]	When possible, recommendations are supported by the best available evidence based on the investigators' collective expertise and review of the medical literature. Recommendations represent the consensus opinion of all investigators who constitute the Board of Directors of The Anticoagulation Forum, an organization dedicated to optimizing anticoagulation care
Managing Oral Anticoagulation Therapy[58]	Written by a diverse, multidisciplinary group of health care providers with clinical experience. Monographs present a systematic, organized, and coordinated model for anticoagulation care. An essential resource for practitioners establishing AMSs to improve the care and outcomes of patients being treated with warfarin

by the AMS, including patient education, systematic INR testing, tracking, follow-up, and good patient communication of results and dosing.[1]

Laboratory devices are available that allow INR measurement from one drop of blood obtained via fingerstick. Use of these devices allows patients to self-test their INR outside the health care setting.[54] The INR results can then be reported to the managing anticoagulation provider for interpretation or for appropriate patients, self-adjustment of the warfarin dose may be possible.[56] Meta-analysis of trials evaluating patient self-testing (PST) and patient self-monitoring (PSM) compared with either management by the community physician or AMS indicate that in appropriately selected patients these strategies can improve the quality of warfarin therapy.[40] Those capable of self-monitoring or self-adjusting therapy had fewer anticoagulation therapy-related complications and in most cases improved INR control. Clearly defined patient selection criteria are required for PST and/or PSM to succeed.[54] Only a few patients taking warfarin are eligible for PST or PSM, and many of these require caregiver assistance; PSM is too demanding for most patients.[40] Fingerstick INR monitoring is more expensive than determination of the INR from venous blood samples in a well-equipped laboratory.[56] In addition, PST and PSM generally involve INR testing at a frequency 2 to 4 times greater than INR testing from venous blood samples, further increasing the cost of therapy.[40] The upfront cost of acquiring the device is prohibitive for some patients, although reimbursement from Medicare is available for eligible patients in the United States. Self-monitoring does offer increased autonomy and convenience for appropriately selected patients who travel frequently.[40]

SUMMARY

Good quality evidence and numerous resources are available to clinicians interested in improving the quality of anticoagulation therapy received by their patients. Consensus guidelines with specific recommendations have been published by various professional organizations (**Table 1**). Although warfarin has been the mainstay of oral anticoagulation therapy for decades, evidence-based methods for improving the quality of warfarin therapy remain underused and, in general, the care of patients receiving warfarin can be improved. In a recent survey, only 6% of primary care physicians and 2% of specialists acknowledged having problems with warfarin dosing, yet warfarin therapy remains generally suboptimally managed and broadly underused.[1,57] The arrival of new anticoagulants that do not require routine laboratory monitoring and lack the significant dietary and drug interaction potential of warfarin is an important evolutionary step in the management of thromboembolic disease. However, it will be years before the efficacy and long-term safety of these new agents are adequately defined. For patients who are able to achieve stable INR control, warfarin remains an important therapeutic option, delivering similar clinical outcomes at a fraction of the cost to the health care system.

REFERENCES

1. Ansell J, Hirsh J, Hylek E, et al. Pharmacology and management of the vitamin K antagonists: American College of Chest Physicians Evidence-Based Clinical Practice Guidelines (8th edition). Chest 2008;133(6 Suppl):160S–98S.
2. Partington SL, Abid S, Teo K, et al. Pre-admission warfarin use in patients with acute ischemic stroke and atrial fibrillation: the appropriate use and barriers to oral anticoagulant therapy. Thromb Res 2007;120(5):663–9.
3. Garcia D, Libby E, Crowther MA. The new oral anticoagulants. Blood 2010; 115(1):15–20.
4. Garcia D. Novel anticoagulants and the future of anticoagulation. Thromb Res 2009;123(Suppl 4):S50–5.
5. Schulman S, Kearon C, Kakkar AK, et al. Dabigatran versus warfarin in the treatment of acute venous thromboembolism. N Engl J Med 2009;361(24):2342–52.
6. Connolly SJ, Ezekowitz MD, Yusuf S, et al. Dabigatran versus warfarin in patients with atrial fibrillation. N Engl J Med 2009;361(12):1139–51.
7. Witt DM, Delate T, Clark NP, et al. Outcomes and predictors of very stable INR control during chronic anticoagulation therapy. Blood 2009;114(5):952–6.
8. Witt DM, Delate T, Clark NP, et al. Twelve-month outcomes and predictors of very stable INR control in prevalent warfarin users. J Thromb Haemost 2010;8:744–9.
9. Wan Y, Heneghan C, Perera R, et al. Anticoagulation control and prediction of adverse events in patients with atrial fibrillation: a systematic review. Circ Cardiovasc Qual Outcomes 2008;1(2):84–91.
10. Singer DE, Chang Y, Fang MC, et al. The net clinical benefit of warfarin anticoagulation in atrial fibrillation. Ann Intern Med 2009;151(5):297–305.
11. Garcia DA, Witt DM, Hylek E, et al. Delivery of optimized anticoagulant therapy: consensus statement from the anticoagulation forum. Ann Pharmacother 2008; 42(7):979–88.
12. Beyth RJ, Quinn LM, Landefeld CS. Prospective evaluation of an index for predicting the risk of major bleeding in outpatients treated with warfarin. Am J Med 1998;105(2):91–9.
13. Shireman TI, Mahnken JD, Howard PA, et al. Development of a contemporary bleeding risk model for elderly warfarin recipients. Chest 2006;130(5):1390–6.
14. Barcellona D, Contu P, Marongiu F. Patient education and oral anticoagulant therapy. Haematologica 2002;87(10):1081–6.
15. Wofford JL, Wells MD, Singh S. Best strategies for patient education about anticoagulation with warfarin: a systematic review. BMC Health Serv Res 2008;8:40.

16. Newall F, Monagle P, Johnston L. Patient understanding of warfarin therapy: a review of education strategies. Hematology 2005;10(6):437–42.

17. Zeolla MM, Brodeur MR, Dominelli A, et al. Development and validation of an instrument to determine patient knowledge: the oral anticoagulation knowledge test. Ann Pharmacother 2006;40(4):633–8.

18. Kovacs MJ, Rodger M, Anderson DR, et al. Comparison of 10-mg and 5-mg warfarin initiation nomograms together with low-molecular-weight heparin for outpatient treatment of acute venous thromboembolism. A randomized, double-blind, controlled trial. Ann Intern Med 2003;138(9):714–9.

19. Crowther MA, Ginsberg JB, Kearon C, et al. A randomized trial comparing 5-mg and 10-mg warfarin loading doses. Arch Intern Med 1999;159(1): 46–8.

20. O'Connell MB, Kowal PR, Allivato CJ, et al. Evaluation of warfarin initiation regimens in elderly inpatients. Pharmacotherapy 2000;20(8):923–30.

21. Siguret V, Gouin I, Debray M, et al. Initiation of warfarin therapy in elderly medical inpatients: a safe and accurate regimen. Am J Med 2005;118(2):137–42.

22. Wadelius M, Chen LY, Lindh JD, et al. The largest prospective warfarin-treated cohort supports genetic forecasting. Blood 2009;113(4):784–92.

23. Klein TE, Altman RB, Eriksson N, et al. Estimation of the warfarin dose with clinical and pharmacogenetic data. N Engl J Med 2009;360(8):753–64.

24. Kangelaris KN, Bent S, Nussbaum RL, et al. Genetic testing before anticoagulation? A systematic review of pharmacogenetic dosing of warfarin. J Gen Intern Med 2009;24(5):656–64.

25. Wilson SE, Costantini L, Crowther MA. Paper-based dosing algorithms for maintenance of warfarin anticoagulation. J Thromb Thrombolysis 2007;23(3): 195–8.

26. Wells PS, Le GG, Tierney S, et al. Practical application of the 10-mg warfarin initiation nomogram. Blood Coagul Fibrinolysis 2009;20(6):403–8.

27. Rose AJ, Ozonoff A, Berlowitz DR, et al. Warfarin dose management affects INR control. J Thromb Haemost 2009;7(1):94–101.

28. Banet GA, Waterman AD, Milligan PE, et al. Warfarin dose reduction vs watchful waiting for mild elevations in the international normalized ratio. Chest 2003; 123(2):499–503.

29. Schulman S, Melinyshyn A, Ennis D, et al. Single-dose adjustment versus no adjustment of warfarin in stably anticoagulated patients with an occasional international normalized ratio (INR) out of range. Thromb Res 2010;125:393–7.

30. Clark NP, Witt DM, Delate T, et al. Thromboembolic consequences of subtherapeutic anticoagulation in patients stabilized on warfarin therapy: the low INR study. Pharmacotherapy 2008;28(8):960–7.

31. Crowther MA, Ageno W, Garcia D, et al. Oral vitamin K versus placebo to correct excessive anticoagulation in patients receiving warfarin: a randomized trial. Ann Intern Med 2009;150(5):293–300.

32. Poller L, Keown M, Ibrahim S, et al. An international multicenter randomized study of computer-assisted oral anticoagulant dosage vs. medical staff dosage. J Thromb Haemost 2008;6(6):935–43.

33. Poller L, Keown M, Ibrahim S, et al. A multicentre randomised assessment of the DAWN AC computer-assisted oral anticoagulant dosage program. Thromb Haemost 2009;101(3):487–94.

34. Poller L, Keown M, Ibrahim S, et al. A multicentre randomised clinical endpoint study of PARMA 5 computer-assisted oral anticoagulant dosage. Br J Haematol 2008;143(2):274–83.

35. Poller L, Shiach CR, MacCallum PK, et al. Multicentre randomised study of computerised anticoagulant dosage. European Concerted Action on Anticoagulation. Lancet 1998;352(9139):1505–9.
36. Fitzmaurice DA, Hobbs FD, Murray ET, et al. Oral anticoagulation management in primary care with the use of computerized decision support and near-patient testing: a randomized, controlled trial. Arch Intern Med 2000;160(15):2343–8.
37. Mitra R, Marciello MA, Brain C, et al. Efficacy of computer-aided dosing of warfarin among patients in a rehabilitation hospital. Am J Phys Med Rehabil 2005;84(6):423–7.
38. Fuster V, Ryden LE, Cannom DS, et al. ACC/AHA/ESC 2006 guidelines for the management of patients with atrial fibrillation: a report of the American College of Cardiology/American Heart Association Task Force on practice guidelines and the European Society of Cardiology Committee for practice guidelines (writing committee to revise the 2001 guidelines for the management of patients with atrial fibrillation): developed in collaboration with the European Heart Rhythm Association and the Heart Rhythm Society. Circulation 2006;114(7):e257–354.
39. Fitzmaurice DA. Oral anticoagulation should be managed in the community with treatment aimed at standard therapeutic targets and increased recall intervals. J Thromb Haemost 2008;6(10):1645–6.
40. Heneghan C, onso-Coello P, Garcia-Alamino JM, et al. Self-monitoring of oral anticoagulation: a systematic review and meta-analysis. Lancet 2006;367(9508): 404–11.
41. Lidstone V, Janes S, Stross P. INR: intervals of measurement can safely extend to 14 weeks. Clin Lab Haematol 2000;22:291–3.
42. Rose AJ, Ozonoff A, Henault LE, et al. Warfarin for atrial fibrillation in community-based practise. J Thromb Haemost 2008;6(10):1647–54.
43. Guidelines on oral anticoagulation: third edition. Br J Haematol 1998;101(2): 374–87.
44. Holbrook AM, Pereira JA, Labiris R, et al. Systematic overview of warfarin and its drug and food interactions. Arch Intern Med 2005;165(10):1095–106.
45. Hirsh J, Fuster V, Ansell J, et al. American Heart Association/American College of Cardiology Foundation guide to warfarin therapy. J Am Coll Cardiol 2003;41(9): 1633–52.
46. Ahmed A, Stephens JC, Kaus CA, et al. Impact of preemptive warfarin dose reduction on anticoagulation after initiation of trimethoprim-sulfamethoxazole or levofloxacin. J Thromb Thrombolysis 2008;26(1):44–8.
47. Lu Y, Won KA, Nelson BJ, et al. Characteristics of the amiodarone-warfarin interaction during long-term follow-up. Am J Health Syst Pharm 2008;65(10):947–52.
48. Lee CR, Thrasher KA. Difficulties in anticoagulation management during coadministration of warfarin and rifampin. Pharmacotherapy 2001;21(10):1240–6.
49. Johnson SG, Witt DM, Eddy TR, et al. Warfarin and antiplatelet combination use among commercially insured patients enrolled in an anticoagulation management service. Chest 2007;131(5):1500–7.
50. Johnson SG, Rogers K, Delate T, et al. Outcomes associated with combined antiplatelet and anticoagulant therapy. Chest 2008;133(4):948–54.
51. de Assis MC, Rabelo ER, Avila CW, et al. Improved oral anticoagulation after a dietary vitamin K-guided strategy: a randomized controlled trial. Circulation 2009;120(12):1115–22, 3.
52. Schurgers LJ, Shearer MJ, Hamulyak K, et al. Effect of vitamin K intake on the stability of oral anticoagulant treatment: dose-response relationships in healthy subjects. Blood 2004;104(9):2682–9.

53. Sconce E, Avery P, Wynne H, et al. Vitamin K supplementation can improve stability of anticoagulation for patients with unexplained variability in response to warfarin. Blood 2007;109(6):2419–23.

54. Ansell J, Jacobson A, Levy J, et al. Guidelines for implementation of patient self-testing and patient self-management of oral anticoagulation. International consensus guidelines prepared by International Self-Monitoring Association for Oral Anticoagulation. Int J Cardiol 2005;99(1):37–45.

55. van WC, Jennings A, Oake N, et al. Effect of study setting on anticoagulation control: a systematic review and metaregression. Chest 2006;129(5):1155–66.

56. Levi M, de Peuter OR, Kamphuisen PW. Management strategies for optimal control of anticoagulation in patients with atrial fibrillation. Semin Thromb Hemost 2009;35(6):560–7.

57. Nieuwlaat R, Barker L, Kim YK, et al. Underuse of evidence-based warfarin dosing methods for atrial fibrillation patients. Thromb Res 2010;125:e128–31.

58. Ansell JE, Oertel LB, Wittkowsky AK. Managing oral anticoagulation therapy. 3rd edition. St Louis (MO): Wolters Kluwer/Facts & Comparisons; 2009.

Oral Xa Inhibitors

Erica Romualdi, MD, Walter Ageno, MD*

KEYWORDS

- Oral anticoagulants • Factor Xa inhibitors • Rivaroxaban
- Apixaban • Edoxaban • Betrixaban

The approach to the development of new anticoagulants as alternatives to heparins and vitamin K antagonists (VKAs) has been guided by the requirement for convenient administration with predictable pharmacokinetics (PK), pharmacodynamics (PD), and a wide therapeutic window that permits fixed dosing without requiring coagulation monitoring. Research has focused in particular on targeting thrombin and factor Xa (FXa), which are common to the intrinsic and extrinsic coagulation pathways. Thus, thrombin inhibitors act to prevent fibrin formation as well as inhibit thrombin-mediated activation of factors V, VIII, XI, and XIII and platelets. Inhibitors of FXa act at an earlier stage in the cascade. They inhibit free and prothrombinase-bound FXa and are also able to inhibit clot-associated FXa, thus preventing clot-associated FXa from activating prothrombin.[1]

After the development of parenteral direct thrombin inhibitors, such as lepirudin or bivalirudin, ximelagatran was the first direct orally available direct thrombin inhibitor. Ximelagatran was withdrawn in 2006 after concerns about liver toxicity. The oral direct thrombin inhibitor, dabigatran etexilate, has recently been approved for use in the European Union and Canada for thromboprophylaxis after total hip replacement surgery (THR) and total knee replacement surgery (TKR) and is currently in an advanced stage of development for other indications. Fondaparinux, a parenteral indirect FXa inhibitor, was the first drug to prove the efficacy of selective FXa inhibition in the prevention and treatment of thromboembolic disease. Several oral FXa inhibitors are now under investigation for the prevention and treatment of thromboembolic disorders, of which rivaroxaban and apixaban are in the most advanced stage of development.

The aim of this review is to provide an overview of the more advanced oral, direct FXa inhibitors and to briefly describe the results of the completed studies.

RIVAROXABAN

Rivaroxaban (BAY 59-7939) is a potent and selective oral FXa inhibitor with a particular chemical structure in its active-site binding region that plays a role in the oral absorption of the drug, with a relatively high bioavailability (nearly 80%).[2] Rivaroxaban has

Department of Clinical Medicine, Research Center on Thromboembolic Disorders and on Antithrombotic Therapies, University of Insubria, U.O. Medicina I, Ospedale di Circolo, Viale Borri 56, Varese 21100, Italy
* Corresponding author. U.O. Medicina I, Ospedale di Circolo, Viale Borri 56, Varese 21100, Italy.
E-mail address: agewal@yahoo.com

Hematol Oncol Clin N Am 24 (2010) 727–737
doi:10.1016/j.hoc.2010.05.006
0889-8588/10/$ – see front matter © 2010 Elsevier Inc. All rights reserved.

a rapid onset of action with predictable, dose proportional PK and PD.[3] Plasma levels of the drug peak after 3 to 4 hours, with a mean half-life ranging from 5 to 9 hours in young individuals and from 11 to 13 hours in the elderly.[4] The main route of excretion is renal, but the drug is also excreted via the fecal/biliary route.[5] Phase I studies demonstrated that gender and body weight did not have a clinically relevant influence on the PK and PD of rivaroxaban in healthy subjects, suggesting that this drug could be administered at a fixed dose in any patient.[6,7] Coadministration with food intake only minimally increases peak plasma concentrations of rivaroxaban,[5] and only a few potential interactions with other drugs have been shown.[8] Rivaroxaban is metabolized in the liver by cythocrome and noncythocrome mechanisms[4] and more than 30% of the drug is excreted in the feces as unchanged drug. Because this phenomenon is, at least in part, mediated by P-glycoprotein, drugs that concomitantly act as strong inhibitors of cytochrome CYP3A4 and P-glycoprotein, such as azole antifungal and HIV-protease inhibitors,[5,9] significantly interfere with the metabolism of rivaroxaban and increase its plasma concentration.

Rivaroxaban for the Prevention of Venous Thromboembolism

In phase II, dose finding studies, rivaroxaban was compared with the low molecular weight heparin (LMWH), enoxaparin, for the prevention of venous thromboembolism (VTE) in patients undergoing THR and TKR;[10–12] in two studies, rivaroxaban was administered twice a day, with a total daily dose ranging from 5 to 60 mg,[10,11] and in a subsequent study,[12] rivaroxaban was given once a day, with a dosage ranging from 5 to 40 mg. Overall, rivaroxaban was well tolerated by the patients, and daily doses between 5 and 20 mg showed efficacy and tolerability that were similar to those of enoxaparin; major bleeding rates increased only with higher doses of rivaroxaban. On the basis of these results, the 10-mg dose administered once daily was selected for subsequent phase III studies. Based on the results of phase I studies[6,7] and of phase II studies, no dose adjustments according to age, body weight, or gender were considered necessary. Rivaroxaban showed the potential to offer clinicians the option of an oral compound that can be administered at a fixed, unmonitored, once-daily dose. The Regulation of Coagulation in Major Orthopedic Surgery Reducing the Risk of DVT and PE (RECORD) program comprised four phase III studies in which rivaroxaban was compared with enoxaparin for the prevention of VTE in more than 12,500 patients undergoing THR and TKR.[13–16]

In RECORD 2,[13] patients undergoing THR were randomized to oral rivaroxaban (10 mg once daily for 35 [±4] days; extended prophylaxis) or to subcutaneous enoxaparin (40 mg once daily for 12 [±2] days; short-term prophylaxis); in RECORD 1,[14] rivaroxaban and enoxaparin, at the same dosages as in RECORD 2, were administered for 35 (±4) days (extended prophylaxis) in patients undergoing THR. In RECORD 3[15] and RECORD 4,[16] rivaroxaban and enoxaparin were administered to patients undergoing TKR for 12 (±2) days, as was recommended by the American College of Chest Physicians guidelines at the time when the studies were planned (2004 guidelines).[17] RECORD 3[15] was conducted primarily in Europe and patients, according to the European standard of practice, received enoxaparin (40 mg once daily) beginning the evening before surgery. Conversely, RECORD 4[16] was conducted primarily in North America and enoxaparin (30 mg twice-daily) was started 12 to 24 hours after surgery according to the standard of practice. In all four studies, rivaroxaban (10 mg once daily) was started 6 to 8 hours after surgery.

Efficacy and safety endpoints were identical in all trials. The primary efficacy endpoint was represented by the occurrence of total VTEs, defined as any deep vein thrombosis (DVT), nonfatal pulmonary embolism (PE), and all-cause mortality.

Secondary efficacy outcomes included major VTEs (ie, proximal DVT, nonfatal PE, or death related to VTE) and symptomatic VTE. The main safety endpoint was major bleeding occurring after the first blinded dose and until up to 2 days after the last dose of study medication. Major bleeding was defined as bleeding that was fatal or involved a critical organ or required reoperation or as clinically overt bleeding outside the surgical site that was associated with a decrease in the hemoglobin level of greater than or equal to 2 g/dL or requiring an infusion of greater than or equal to 2 units of blood. Also assessed were nonmajor bleeding, including hemorrhagic wound complications (excessive wound hematoma or bleeding at the surgical site), other adverse events, including liver toxicity and cardiovascular events, and death.

In RECORD 2,[13] the incidence of the primary efficacy outcome was significantly reduced from 9.3% in the group of patients receiving short-term enoxaparin to 2.0% in the group of patients receiving long-term rivaroxaban (relative risk reduction [RRR] 79%, $P<.0001$). The incidence of major and symptomatic VTEs were also significantly reduced from 5.1% to 0.6% (RRR 88%, $P<.0001$), and 1.2% to 0.2% (RRR 80%, $P = .004$), respectively.

In RECORD 1,[14] total VTEs were reduced from 3.7% in the group of patients receiving enoxaparin to 1.1% in the group of patients receiving rivaroxaban (RRR 70%, $P<.001$), and the incidence of major VTEs was reduced from 2.0% to 0.2%, respectively (RRR 88%, $P<.001$). Symptomatic VTEs occurred in 0.5% in the enoxaparin group and in 0.3% of patients in the rivaroxaban group.

In RECORD 3,[15] all primary and secondary efficacy endpoints were reduced with the use of rivaroxaban. Total VTEs were reduced from 18.9% in the group of patients receiving enoxaparin to 9.6% in the group of patients receiving rivaroxaban (RRR 49%, $P<.0001$), major VTEs from 2.6% to 1.0% (RRR 62%, $P = .010$), and symptomatic VTEs from 2.0% to 0.7%, respectively (RRR 66%, $P = .005$).

Finally, RECORD 4[16] demonstrated that rivaroxaban was more effective than enoxaparin administered at a dosage of 30 mg once daily for the prevention of total VTEs (rivaroxaban 6.9% vs enoxaparin 10.1%, RRR 31%, $P = .012$). The rates of major VTEs and symptomatic VTEs with rivaroxaban and enoxaparin were 1.2% versus 2.0% and 0.7% versus 1.2%, respectively.

In all RECORD studies rivaroxaban showed a similar rate of major bleeding events and clinically relevant nonmajor bleeding events, when compared with enoxaparin. This was also supported by the absence of laboratory signs of compromised liver function attributable to rivaroxaban. The results of the RECORD studies are summarized in **Table 1**.

A clinical trial evaluating rivaroxaban for the prevention of VTE in high-risk medical patients, the Multicenter, Randomized, Parallel Group Efficacy and Safety Study for the Prevention of Venous Thromboembolism in Hospitalized Medically Ill Patients Comparing Rivaroxaban with Enoxaparin (MAGELLAN) study, is currently ongoing. In MAGELLAN, a double-blind, double-dummy study, patients are randomized to receive rivaroxaban administered at a dosage of 10 mg once daily for 35 (±4) days or enoxaparin 40 mg once daily for 10 (±4) days.

Rivaroxaban for the Treatment of VTE

In addition to thromboprophylaxis, rivaroxaban is also being evaluated for the treatment of VTE. Two phase II, dose finding studies compared rivaroxaban administered at total daily doses ranging from 20 to 60 mg with standard therapy with LMWH followed by oral VKAs.[18,19] Based on the positive results of these studies, three phase III clinical trials aimed to assess the acute phase and the long term treatment of DVT and PE have been initiated. Rivaroxaban dosages of 15 mg twice daily for 3 weeks followed by 20 mg once

Table 1
Results of RECORD studies

Study	Patient Group (n)	% Primary Efficacy Endpoint (Composite of Any DVT, Nonfatal PE, and All-Cause Mortality)	% Relative Risk Reduction (P value)	% Primary Safety Endpoint: Major Bleeding (Number)[e]
RECORD1[a,14] Extended prophylaxis with oral rivaroxaban versus extended sc enoxaparin	THA (4541)			
Rivaroxaban (10 mg od)		1.1 (18/1595)	70 (P<.001)	0.3 (6/2209)
Enoxaparin (40 mg od)		3.7 (58/1558)		0.1 (2/2224)
RECORD2[b,13] Extended prophylaxis with oral rivaroxaban versus short-term sc enoxaparin	THA (2509)			
Rivaroxaban (10 mg od)		2.0 (17/864)	79 (P<.001)	<0.1 (1/1228)
Enoxaparin (40 mg od)		9.3 (81/869)		<0.1 (1/1229)
RECORD3[c,15] Thromboprophylaxis with oral rivaroxaban versus sc enoxaparin	TKA (2531)			
Rivaroxaban (10 mg od)		9.6 (79/824)	49 (P<.001)	0.6 (7/1220)
Enoxaparin (40 mg od)		18.9 (166/878)		0.5 (6/1239)
RECORD4[d,16] Thromboprophylaxis with oral rivaroxaban versus sc enoxaparin	TKA (3148)			
Rivaroxaban (10 mg od)		6.9 (67/965)	31 (P = .012)	0.7 (10/1526)
Enoxaparin (30 mg bid)		10.1 (97/959)		0.3 (4/1508)

a Oral, once-daily rivaroxaban (10 mg), started 6–8 hours after surgery, versus sc once-daily enoxaparin (40 mg), started the evening before surgery. Both regimens continued for 36 (±6) days.

b Oral, once-daily rivaroxaban (10 mg), started 6–8 hours after surgery, for 35 (±4) days, versus sc once-daily enoxaparin (40 mg), started the evening before surgery, continued for 12 (±2) days, followed by placebo.

c Oral, once-daily rivaroxaban (10 mg), started 6–8 hours after surgery for 12 (±2) days, versus sc once-daily enoxaparin (40 mg), started the evening before surgery, continued for 12 (±2) days, followed by placebo.

d Oral, once-daily rivaroxaban (10 mg), started 6–8 hours after surgery for 12 (±2) days, versus sc twice-daily enoxaparin (30 mg), started the evening before surgery, continued for 12 (±2) days, followed by placebo.

e Major bleeding was defined as bleeding that was fatal, involved a critical organ, or required reoperation or clinically overt bleeding outside the surgical site that was associated with a decrease in the hemoglobin level of ≥2 g/d or requiring an infusion of ≥2 units of blood.

daily are used in the ongoing EINSTEIN-DVT and EINSTEIN-PE studies. These studies enroll patients with objectively confirmed, symptomatic DVT or PE who are randomized to treatment with rivaroxaban alone or with LMWH and VKAs for a total period of 3 to 12 months. The EINSTEIN-Extension study treats patients with rivaroxaban (20 mg once daily) or placebo after 6 to 12 months of treatment with VKAs or rivaroxaban. This study is completed, and the results have been presented at the American Society of Hematology meeting in December 2009.[20] The primary efficacy outcome was the recurrence of symptomatic VTE and the principal safety outcome was the occurrence of major bleeding. A total of 1197 patients were randomized between February 2007 and May 2009. The intention-to-treat population consisted of 602 rivaroxaban and 594 placebo patients. The mean duration of study treatment was 190 days in both groups. During the treatment period, symptomatic recurrent VTE events occurred in 42 (7.1%) patients treated with placebo and in 8 (1.3%) patients treated with rivaroxaban (hazard ratio, 0.18; 95% CI, 0.09–0.39). After stopping the study medication, 6 (1.0%) symptomatic recurrent VTE events occurred in both groups during the 1-month observational period of follow-up. No major bleeding events were documented in the group of patients treated with placebo; 4 (0.7%) major bleeding events occurred in the rivaroxaban group ($P = .106$). None of these bleeding events was fatal or occurred in a critical site. Clinically relevant nonmajor bleeding occurred in 7 (1.2%) and in 32 (5.4%) patients randomized to placebo and rivaroxaban, respectively. Two (0.3%) patients in the placebo group and 1 (0.2%) patient in the rivaroxaban group died. No patients had documented liver toxicity defined as an alanine aminotransferase rise above 3 times the upper limit of normal combined with a total bilirubin above 2 times the upper limit of normal. Thus, the fixed dose of rivaroxaban (20 mg once daily) administered for the long-term secondary prevention of VTE resulted in a significant reduction in the recurrence of VTE as compared with no treatment, and, most of all, active therapy with rivaroxaban was not associated with an increased incidence of major bleeding events.

Rivaroxaban for the Prevention and Treatment of Arterial Thrombosis

The 20-mg once-daily dose of rivaroxaban was also chosen in the Randomized, Double-Blind Study Comparing Once Daily Oral Rivaroxaban with Adjusted-Dose Oral Warfarin for the Prevention of Stroke in Subjects with Non-Valvular Atrial Fibrillation (ROCKET AF) study, a phase III study on the long-term prevention of stroke in patients with atrial fibrillation (www.clinicaltrials.gov; NCT00403767). In the ROCKET AF study, patients with high-risk, nonvalvular atrial fibrillation are randomized to treatment with warfarin, administered to achieve an international normalized ratio (INR) range between 2.0 and 3.0, or to treatment with rivaroxaban. In this study, a lower dose of rivaroxaban (ie, 15 mg once daily) is administered to patients with a creatinine clearance of between 30 and 49 mL per minute. The enrollment phase of the ROCKET AF study is now completed, and the results should be available by the end of 2010.

Finally, rivaroxaban was also tested in patients with acute coronary syndrome (ACS) in a phase II study.[21] The Rivaroxaban in Combination with Aspirin Alone or with Aspirin and Thienopyridine in Subjects with Acute Coronary Syndromes (ATLAS ACS-TIMI 46) trial is a randomized, double-blind, placebo-controlled dose escalation study created to assess the safety and efficacy of rivaroxaban in patients with ACS. In this study patients receiving aspirin (stratum 1) or aspirin plus thienopyridine (stratum 2), after the acute coronary event, were randomized to receive placebo or rivaroxaban, administered at a total daily dose (range, 5–20 mg) given once or twice daily. The primary safety endpoint was clinically relevant bleeding; the primary efficacy endpoint was the time to the first episode of death, myocardial infarction, stroke, or severe recurrent ischemia requiring revascularization. Clinically relevant bleeding occurred in a dose-dependent manner: compared with placebo, rivaroxaban was associated with a significant increase in bleeding rates, with hazard ratios (HRs) ranging from 2.21 (CI, 1.25–3.91) for the 5-mg dose to 5.06 (3.45–7.42) for the 20-mg dose. The increase in bleeding across doses was apparent in both strata, but the absolute rates of clinically relevant bleeding were lower in stratum 1 than in stratum 2. Compared with placebo, treatment with rivaroxaban resulted in a hazard ratio (HR) of 3.96 (CI, 1.40–11.23) for clinically relevant bleeding in stratum 1 and of 3.66 (CI, 2.54–5.27) in stratum 2. Across the entire population, rates of the primary efficacy endpoint were 5.5% in the group receiving rivaroxaban and 7.0% in the group receiving placebo (HR 0.79; CI, 0.60–1.05), with this risk reduction being statistically significant in stratum 1 (HR 0.53; CI, 0.33–0.84), but not in stratum 2 (HR 0.99; CI, 0.9–1.42). On the basis of these observations, a larger, phase III clinical trial was then planned with the aim to analyze the efficacy of rivaroxaban at the doses of 2.5 mg and 5 mg administered twice daily in ACS patients (www.clinicaltrials.gov; NCT00809965).

APIXABAN

Apixaban is an oral active FXa inhibitor derived from razaxaban (an aminobenzisoxazole that binds to the active site of FXa with high affinity), with superior pharmacologic properties.[22] It is a small molecule able to inhibit in a selective and reversible manner the active site of free and prothrombinase-bound FXa.[1] Preclinical studies demonstrate that apixaban has an oral bioavailability of more than 50%: its plasma peak is achieved in approximately 3 hours and its half-life is approximately 12 hours.[23] The drug is absorbed in the gastrointestinal tract, is metabolized in the liver by cytochrome-dependent and -independent mechanisms, and is eliminated through the renal and the fecal routes.[5] Food does not interfere with its absorption, so that the drug generates a predictable anticoagulation effect.[5] The results of in vitro studies suggest that the metabolic drug-drug interaction potential between apixaban and coadministered drugs is low.[24] Interaction studies show that coadministration of apixaban with digoxin has no significant effect.[5]

Apixaban for the Prevention of VTE

Apixaban was first tested in a phase IIb, dose finding study, Apixaban Prophylaxis in Patients Undergoing Total Knee Replacement Surgery (APROPOS), and was compared with enoxaparin (30 mg twice a day) or warfarin (INR range, 1.8–3.0) for the prevention of VTE in patients undergoing TKR. Apixaban was administered at total daily doses given once daily or twice a day (range, 5–20 mg).[25] Based on the results of the APROPOS study, a 2.5-mg twice-daily dose was chosen for the phase III program, based on three randomized controlled trials in patients undergoing THR and TKR.

In one randomized, phase III study (Apixaban Dose Orally vs Anticoagulant with Enoxaparin [ADVANCE]-1 study) apixaban was compared with enoxaparin for the prevention of VTE in patients undergoing TKR.[26] In this study, patients were randomized to receive apixaban (2.5 mg twice a day) or enoxaparin (30 mg twice a day). Both medications were started postoperatively (12 to 24 hours after surgery) and continued for 12 ($\pm$2) days, until mandatory bilateral venography. The primary efficacy outcome was a composite of asymptomatic and symptomatic DVT, fatal and nonfatal PE, and death from any cause during treatment. The rate of the primary efficacy outcome was 9.0% with apixaban as compared with 8.8% with enoxaparin (relative risk 1.02; 95% CI, 0.78–1.32). Although substantially equivalent to enoxaparin in efficacy, apixaban did not meet the prespecified criterion of noninferiority as compared with twice-daily administration of enoxaparin. Alternatively, apixaban showed a greater safety profile, with the composite incidence of major bleeding and clinically relevant nonmajor bleeding being 2.9% with apixaban and 4.3% with enoxaparin ($P = .03$). The results of the ADVANCE 2 study were presented at the International Society on Thrombosis and Haemostasis meeting in Boston.[27] In this study, apixaban (2.5 mg twice a day) administered for 12 (±2) days was compared with enoxaparin administered according to the European standard regimens of 40 mg once daily started preoperatively in patients undergoing TKR. In ADVANCE 2, the primary efficacy endpoint, which was the same as in ADVANCE 1, was significantly reduced from 24.4% in the group receiving enoxaparin to 15.1% in the group receiving apixaban (relative risk 0.62; CI, 0.51–0.74). The secondary efficacy outcome, including proximal DVT-, PE-, and VTE-related death, was also significantly reduced from 2.2% to 1.1%, respectively (relative risk 0.50; CI, 0.26–0.97). No statistically significant difference between the two drugs was observed in the primary safety outcome combining major and clinically relevant nonmajor bleeding, with an incidence of 3.5% in the group receiving apixaban and 4.8% in the group receiving enoxaparin. No signs of liver toxicity were detected in either group. Finally, the ADVANCE 3 study comparing apixaban (2.5 mg twice a day) and enoxaparin (40 mg once daily) for long-term prophylaxis in patients undergoing THR is currently under way (www.clinicaltrials.gov; NCT00423319). The results of ADVANCE 1 and 2 studies are summarized in **Table 2**.

In high-risk medical patients, the ongoing Apixaban for the Prevention of Thrombosis-Related Events in Patients with Acute Medical Illness (ADOPT) is comparing apixaban (2.5 mg twice a day) administered for 30 days with enoxaparin (40 mg once daily) given for at least a week (www.clinicaltrials.gov; NCT00457002). Another study is evaluating apixaban for the prevention of VTE in patients with metastatic cancer (www.clinicaltrials.gov; NCT00412984).

Apixaban for the Treatment of VTE

Apixaban has been assessed for the treatment of DVT in a dose finding study (Botticelli DVT study);[28] in this setting, patients were randomized to receive apixaban (5 mg twice a day, 10 mg twice a day, or 20 mg once daily) or LMWH/VKA. The primary efficacy outcome, defined as the composite of symptomatic recurrent VTE and asymptomatic deterioration in the thrombotic burden as assessed by repeat bilateral compression ultrasonography and perfusion lung scan, occurred in 4.7% of patients treated with apixaban and in 4.2% of LMWH/VKA-treated patients. No dose effect was observed across apixaban doses. The principal safety outcome, defined as the composite of major and clinically relevant nonmajor bleeding, occurred in 7.3% of the apixaban-treated patients and in 7.9% of LMWH/VKA-treated patients. There was no evidence of liver toxicity. On the basis of this study, phase III studies (Apixaban After the Initial Management of Pulmonary Embolism and Deep Vein Thrombosis with First Line Therapy [AMPLIFY] and AMPLIFY extension), testing apixaban (at dosages of 10 mg and 5 mg twice daily) are now under way (www.clinicaltrials.gov; NCT00633893 and NCT00643201).

Apixaban for the Prevention and Treatment of Arterial Thrombosis

Apixaban for Prevention of Acute Ischemic and Safety Events (APPRAISE) is a phase II clinical trial in which patients with ACS were randomized to 6 months of placebo or to 6 months of apixaban administered at 4 different doses (range, 5–20 mg) on top of standard antiplatelet therapy.[29] The primary outcome of major or clinically relevant nonmajor bleeding was increased in all apixaban-treated patients, and the two higher-dose apixaban arms were prematurely discontinued because of excess total bleeding. The hazard ratios for the primary outcome in the two lower-dose arms were 1.78 (CI, 0.91–3.48) in the 2.5-mg, twice-a-day dose group and 2.45 (CI, 1.31–4.61) in the 10-mg, once-daily group. Both doses resulted in nonsignificantly lower rates of ischemic events when compared with placebo, with hazard ratios of 0.73

Table 2
Results of ADVANCE 1 and 2 studies

Study	Patient Group (n)	% Primary Efficacy Endpoint (Composite of Any DVT, Nonfatal PE, and All-Cause Mortality)	Relative Risk	% Primary Safety Endpoint: Major Bleeding and Clinically Relevant Nonmajor Bleeding[c]
ADVANCE 1[a,26] Thromboprophylaxis with oral apixaban versus sc enoxaparin	TKR (3195)			
Apixaban (2.5 mg bid)		9 (104/1157)	1.02	2.9 (46/1596)
Enoxaparin (30 mg bid)		8.8 (100/1130)	(CI, 0.78–1.32)	4.3 (68/1588)
ADVANCE 2[b,27] Thromboprophylaxis with oral apixaban versus sc enoxaparin	TKR (3057)			
Apixaban (2.5 mg bid)		15.1 (147/976)	0.62	3.5 (53/?)
Enoxaparin (40 mg od)		24.4 (243/997)	(CI, 0.51–0.74)	4.8 (72/?)

[a] Oral, twice-daily apixaban (2.5 mg), started 12–24 hours after surgery, versus sc twice-daily enoxaparin (30 mg), started 12–24 hours after surgery. Both regimens continued for 12 (±2) days.
[b] Oral, twice-daily apixaban, (2.5 mg), started 12–24 hours after surgery, versus sc once-daily enoxaparin (40 mg), started the evening before surgery, continued for 12 (±2) days.
[c] Major bleeding was defined as acute, clinically overt bleeding accompanied by one or more of the following events: a decrease in the hemoglobin level of 2 g/dL or more within a 24-hour period; a transfusion of 2 or more units of packed red cells; bleeding at a critical site (ie, intracranial, intraspinal, intraocular, pericardial, or retroperitoneal); bleeding into the operated joint, requiring an additional operation or intervention; intramuscular bleeding with the compartment syndrome; or fatal bleeding. The definition of clinically relevant nonmajor bleeding included acute, clinically overt bleeding, such as wound hematoma, bruising, or ecchymosis; gastrointestinal bleeding; hemoptysis; hematuria; or epistaxis that did not meet the other criteria for major bleeding.

(CI, 0.44–1.19) and 0.61 (CI, 0.35–1.04), respectively. A phase III clinical trial (APPRAISE-2) comparing apixaban (5 mg twice a day) with placebo in patients with ACS is ongoing (www.clinicaltrials.gov; NCT00831441). Finally, two randomized controlled trials, Apixaban for the Prevention of Stroke in Subjects with Atrial Fibrillation (ARISTOTLE) (www.clinicaltrials.gov; NCT00412984), and Apixaban Versus Acetylsalicylic Acid to Prevent Strokes (AVERROES) (www.clinicaltrials.gov; NCT00496769) are assessing apixaban (5 mg twice a day) for the prevention of stroke in patients with atrial fibrillation. In ARISTOTLE, apixaban is compared with warfarin in patients with at least one additional risk factor; in AVERROES, apixaban is compared with aspirin in patients who are deemed ineligible for VKA treatment.

OTHER FACTOR XA INHIBITORS WITH COMPLETED AND PUBLISHED CLINICAL TRIALS

Betrixaban is another oral direct anti FXa inhibitor with bioavailability of 47% and half-life of 19 hours; it has predictable PD and PK, has minimal interactions with food, and is excreted almost unchanged in bile.[1] This drug was tested for the prevention of VTE in a phase II randomized controlled study in patients undergoing TKR.[30] In the Evaluation of Betrixaban for Prevention of Thromboembolic Events After Total Knee Replacement (EXPERT) study, betrixaban (at a dosage of 15 mg or 40 mg twice a day) was compared with enoxaparin (30 mg subcutaneous twice a day) for 12 (±2) days; VTE incidence was 20% (CI, 11%–31%) for betrixaban (15 mg), 15% (CI, 8%–27%) for betrixaban (40 mg), and 10% (CI, 3%–24%) for enoxaparin.

LY517717 is an oral FXa inhibitor with a half-life of 25 hours and elimination primarily via the gastrointestinal route.[1] In a phase II study, this drug was compared with enoxaparin for the prevention of VTE in patients undergoing TKR or THR.[31] In this study, LY517717 (at doses of 100 mg, 125 mg, and 150 mg) seemed to be not inferior to enoxaparin given at a dose of 40 mg, with a lower rate of major bleeding.

SUMMARY

Several new oral drugs that selectively and directly inhibit FXa seem promising alternatives to existing antithrombotic drugs. All these drugs have a convenient route of administration, can be given in fixed doses, and do not require coagulation monitoring, thanks to their predictable anticoagulant responses and their low potential for food-drug and drug-drug interactions. The favorable results of clinical trials support their potential to change current practice, in particular in the management of patients requiring long-term anticoagulant treatment. Rivaroxaban is the first of this new class of drugs to be approved for the prevention of VTE after elective THR or TKR surgery in the European Union, in Canada, and in several other countries. Although practical advantages are self-evident, translation into daily clinical practice may take some time and only reports from clinical studies over the next months and years will reveal the impact of rivaroxaban as well as of other compounds in earlier stages of development.

Several issues with these novel agents need to be addressed before they are used widely in clinical practice; these include the optimal management of major bleeding complications given the current lack of specific antidotes; the lack of laboratory tests, which can measure their amount of drug present in individual patients; and their cost relative to currently available drugs.

REFERENCES

1. Turpie AGG. Oral direct Factor Xa inhibitors in development for the prevention and treatment of thromboembolic diseases. Arterioscler Thromb Vasc Biol 2007;27:1238–47.
2. Eriksson BI, Quinlan DJ. Oral anticoagulants in development—focus on thromboprophylaxis in patients undergoing orthopedic surgery. Drugs 2006;66(11):1411–29.
3. Kubitza D, Becka M, Voith B, et al. Safety pharmacodynamics and pharmacokinetics of BAY39-7959, an oral direct factor Xa inhibitor. Clin Pharmacol Ther 2005;78:412–21.
4. Eriksson BI, Quinlan DJ, Weitz JI. Comparative pharmacodynamics and pharmacokinetics of oral direct thrombin and factor Xa inhibitors development. Clin Pharmacokinet 2009;48:1–22.
5. Kubitza D, Becka M, Wensing G, et al. Safety pharmacodynamics and pharmacokinetics of BAY39-7959, an oral direct factor Xa inhibitor—after multiple dosing in healthy male subjects. Eur J Clin Pharmacol 2005;61:873–80.

6. Kubitza D, Becka M, Mueck W, et al. The effect of extreme age, and gender, on the pharmacology and tolerability of rivaroxaban—an oral direct Factor Xa inhibitor [abstract 905]. Blood 2006;108.

7. Kubitza D, Becka M, Zuehlsdorf M, et al. Effects of a single dose BAY39-7959—an oral direct factor Xa inhibitor—in subjects with extreme body weight [abstract 1872]. Blood 2005;106.

8. Kubitza D, Haas S. Novel factor Xa inhibitors for the prevention and treatment of thromboembolic diseases. Expert Opin Investig Drugs 2006;15:843–55.

9. European Medicines Agency (EMEA). European public assessment report: Xarelto. Available at: http://www.emea.europa.eu. Accessed February 2010.

10. Turpie AG, Fisher WD, Bauer KA, et al. BAY 59-7939: an oral direct factor Xa inhibitor for the prevention of venous thromboembolism in patients after total knee replacement. A phase II dose ranging study. J Thromb Haemost 2005;3:2479–86.

11. Eriksson BI, Borris L, Dahl OE, et al. Oral direct Factor Xa inhibition with BAY59-7939 for the prevention of venous thromboembolism after total hip replacement. J Thromb Haemost 2006;4:121–8.

12. Eriksson BI, Borris LC, Dahl OE, et al. A once-daily, oral, direct Factor Xa inhibitor, rivaroxaban (BAY59-7939), for thromboprophylaxis after total hip replacement. Circulation 2006;114:2374–81.

13. Kakkar AK, Brenner B, Dahl OE, et al. Extended duration rivaroxaban versus short-term enoxaparin for the prevention of venous thromboembolism after total hip arthroplasty: a double-blind randomized controlled trial. Lancet 2008;372:31–9.

14. Eriksson BI, Borris LC, Friedman RJ, et al. Rivaroxaban versus enoxaparin for thromboprophylaxis after hip arthroplasty. N Engl J Med 2008;358:2765–75.

15. Lassen MR, Ageno W, Borris LC, et al. Rivaroxaban for thromboprophylaxis after total knee arthroplasty. N Engl J Med 2008;358:2776–85.

16. Turpie AG, Lassen MR, Davidson BL, et al. Rivaroxaban versus enoxaparin for thromboprophylaxis after total knee arthroplasty (RECORD 4): a randomized trial. Lancet 2009;373:1673–80.

17. Geerts WH, Pineo GF, Heit JH, et al. Prevention of venous thromboembolism: the Seventh ACCP conference on antithrombotic and thrombolytic therapy. Chest 2004;126:338–400.

18. Agnelli G, Gallus A, Goldhaber S, et al. Treatment of proximal deep venous thrombosis with the oral, direct factor Xa inhibitor rivaroxaban (BAY59-7939)-the ODIXa DVT (oral direct factor Xa inhibitor BAY59-7939 in patients with acute symptomatic deep vein thrombosis) study. Circulation 2007;116(2):180–7.

19. Buller HR, Lensing AW, Prins MH, et al. A dose-ranging study evaluating once-daily oral administration of the factor Xa inhibitor rivaroxaban in the treatment of patients with acute symptomatic deep vein thrombosis: the Einstein-DVT Dose-Ranging Study. Blood 2008;112(6):2242–7.

20. Buller HR. Once daily oral rivaroxaban versus placebo in the long term prevention of recurrent symptomatic venous thromboembolism. The Einstein-Extension study [abstract 2]. Blood 2009;114.

21. Mega JL, Braunwald E, Mohanavelu S, et al. Rivaroxaban versus placebo in patients with acute coronary syndromes (Atlas ACS -TIMI 46): a randomised double blind, phase II trial. Lancet 2009;374:29–38.

22. Weits JI, Bates SM. New anticoagulants. J Thromb Haemost 2005;3:1843–53.

23. Wong PC, Crain EJ, Xin B, et al. Apixaban, an oral, direct and selective factor Xa inhibitor: in vitro, antithrombotic and antihemostatic studies. J Thromb Haemost 2007;6:820–9.

24. Wang L, Zhang D, Raghavan N, et al. In vitro assessment of metabolic drug-drug interaction potential of apixaban through cytochrome P450 phenotyping, inhibition, and induction studies. Drug Metab Dispos 2010;38(3):448–58.

25. Lassen MR, Davidson BL, Gallus A, et al. The efficacy and safety of apixaban, an oral, direct, factor Xa inhibitor, as thromboprophylaxis in patients following total knee replacement. J Thromb Haemost 2007;5:2368–75.

26. Lassen MR, Raskob GE, Gallus A. Apixaban or enoxaparin for the thromboprophylaxis after knee replacement. N Engl J Med 2009;361:594–604.

27. Lassen MR, Gallus AS, Pineo GF, et al. The ADVANCE 2 study: a randomized double blind trial comparing apixaban with enoxaparin for thromboprophylaxis after total knee replacement [abstract LB-MO-005]. J Thromb Haemost 2009; 7(S2).

28. Buller H, Deichman D, Prins M. Efficacy and safety of the oral direct facto Xa inhibitor apixaban for the symptomatic deep vein thrombosis. The Botticelli DVT dose ranging study. J Thromb Haemost 2008;6:1313–8.

29. Alexander JH, Becker RC, Bhatt DL, et al. Apixaban, an oral, direct, selective factor Xa inhibitor, in combination with antiplatelet therapy after acute coronary syndrome: results of the Apixaban for Prevention of Acute Ischemic and Safety Events (APPRAISE) trial. Circulation 2009;119:2877–85.

30. Turpie AG, Bauer KA, Davidson BL, et al. A randomized evaluation of betrixaban, an oral factor Xa inhibitor, for prevention of thromboembolic events after total knee replacement (EXPERT). Thromb Haemost 2009;101(1):68–76.

31. Agnelli G, Haas S, Ginsberg JS, et al. A phase II study of the oral factor Xa inhibitor LY517717 for the prevention of venous thromboembolism after hip or knee replacement. J Thromb Haemost 2007;5:746–53.

Oral IIa Inhibitors

Catherine J. Lee, MD, Gauri Badhwar, DO, Jack E. Ansell, MD*

KEYWORDS

- Dabigatran etexilate • Oral IIa inhibitors
- Venous thromboembolism • Prevention • Thrombin
- Oral anticoagulation

From the early 1940s, the vitamin K antagonists (VKAs; warfarin, phenprocoumon, acenocoumarol) have been the only oral anticoagulants available for the long-term treatment of venous and selected arterial thromboembolic disease. In the last decade, new classes of oral anticoagulants have emerged and undergone extensive study. At present, the oral direct thrombin inhibitors and oral factor Xa inhibitors are the most promising agents and the most advanced in study. Because of their size, structure, and pharmacokinetics, these agents have specific advantages over the VKAs and they may also be suited to replace the heparin anticoagulants for selected conditions. Specifically, they directly inhibit their target enzyme, they are small molecules and can interact with their target in the fibrin clot or prothrombinase complex, respectively; their pharmacokinetics are predictable; and they have few if any drug or food interactions such that monitoring is not required. This article reviews the oral direct thrombin inhibitors and the class of new anticoagulants of which ximelagatran is the first example of an alternative to the VKAs.

XIMELAGATRAN

Ximelagatran (Exanta) was the first oral direct thrombin inhibitor to be developed. Although it was found to be an effective therapy for the prevention and treatment of venous thromboembolism (VTE) and stroke prevention in atrial fibrillation (AF), it was associated with hepatotoxicity and removed from the market in Europe, and was never approved in North America. However, because it served as a template for the study of other direct thrombin inhibitors, it is briefly reviewed here. Ximelagatran, the inactive prodrug for melagatran, has approximately 80 times greater membrane permeability when taken orally, which makes it a rapidly absorbable drug.[1–3] Once absorbed, ximelagatran is converted to melagatran via hydrolysis of the ester group and reduction of the hydroxyl group.[2] It reaches peak plasma levels in 2 to 3 hours, has a half-life of 3 to 5 hours, and is administered as a twice-daily dose drug. Ximelagatran has minimal drug interactions and a predictable response, therefore not

---

Department of Medicine, Lenox Hill Hospital, 6 Black Hall, 100 East 77th Street, New York, NY 10075, USA
* Corresponding author.
E-mail address: jansell@lenoxhill.net

Hematol Oncol Clin N Am 24 (2010) 739–753
doi:10.1016/j.hoc.2010.05.001
0889-8588/10/$ – see front matter © 2010 Elsevier Inc. All rights reserved.

requiring monitoring. Its primary route of excretion is via the kidneys.[2,3] Ximelagatran has been studied for the prevention of venous thromboembolism following major orthopedic surgery, treatment of acute and chronic venous thromboembolism, stroke prevention in AF, and secondary prevention of cardiovascular events after an acute myocardial infarction.[3]

Prevention of Venous Thromboembolism in Orthopedic Surgery

Several phase 3 trials in total hip and knee replacement surgery showed ximelagatran to have excellent efficacy and safety in VTE prevention following orthopedic surgery. The MElagatran for THROmbin inhibition in orthopedic surgery (METHRO) III study of 2800 patients undergoing hip or knee replacement showed that postoperative administration of 3 mg subcutaneous melagatran followed by ximelagatran 24 mg twice a day for 8 to 11 days had an efficacy comparable to enoxaparin initiated preoperatively (total VTE 31% vs 27.3%, respectively; $P = .053$). Rates of severe bleeding between ximelagatran (1.4%; 95% confidence interval [CI], 0.9%–2.2%) and enoxaparin (1.7%; 95% CI, 1.1%–2.5%) did not differ.[3,4] In the expanded prophylaxis evaluation surgery (EXPRESS) study, administration of melagatran 2 mg preoperatively followed by a 3 mg dose postoperatively, and then ximelagatran 24 mg twice a day starting the next day versus preoperative initiation of enoxaparin demonstrated significantly lower rates of proximal deep vein thrombosis (DVT) and pulmonary embolism (PE) (2.3% vs 6.3%, respectively; $P<.001$) and total VTE (20.3% vs 26.6%, respectively; $P<.0014$).[5] However, severe bleeding was greater with melagatran/ximelagatran than with enoxaparin (3.1% vs 1.2%, respectively; $P<.001$).[5]

In a North American trial of 1800 patients undergoing total hip replacement, ximelagatran 24 mg twice a day and enoxaparin 30 mg twice a day, both started postoperatively, failed to meet noninferiority criteria (total VTE 7.9% vs 4.6%, absolute difference, 3.3%; 95% CI, 0.9%–5.7%). Major bleeding events were similar in both groups.[6] In the Exanta Used To Lessen Thrombosis (EXULT) A trial, 1800 patients undergoing total knee replacement surgery received ximelagatran 24 mg or 36 mg twice a day started postoperatively and were compared with postoperative administration of warfarin (adjusted for international normalized ratio [INR] 1.8–3.0). The 36 mg dose of ximelagatran achieved lower rates of VTE and all-cause mortality compared with warfarin (20.3% vs 27.6%, respectively; $P = .003$).[7] Major bleeding occurred in 0.8% of both ximelagatran groups versus 0.7% in the warfarin group. A follow-up study, EXULT B, confirmed the benefit of the higher ximelagatran dose of 36 mg twice daily compared with warfarin (adjusted for INR = 2.5) after total knee replacement in 2300 patients. Total venous thromboembolism and all-cause mortality combined occurred in 22.5% vs 31.9%, respectively ($P<.001$).[3,8]

Stroke Prevention in AF

Stroke prevention with the oral direct thrombin inhibitor ximelagatran compared with warfarin in patients with nonvalvular atrial fibrillation (SPORTIF) III AND SPORTIF V studies compared ximelagatran 36 mg twice a day with warfarin (target INR = 2.5) for prevention of stroke and systemic thromboembolism in more than 7300 patients with nonvalvular AF and additional stroke risk factors. SPORTIF III was a randomized, open-label trial whereas SPORTIF V was blinded.[9] In SPORTIF III, an intention to treat analysis demonstrated an absolute risk reduction of 0.7% (95% CI, −0.1–1.4; $P = .10$) favoring ximelagatran.[10] There was no significant difference in major bleeding. Elevations in alanine aminotransferase (ALT) levels greater than 3 times the upper limit of normal were experienced by 6% of patients receiving ximelagatran compared with 1% of the patients in the warfarin group ($P<.001$),[10] and 3.4% of ximelagatran patients had ALT elevations greater than 5 times the upper limit of normal. Elevations in ALT levels in the ximelagatran group occurred in the first 2 to 6 months of the start of therapy.[10]

In SPORTIF V (3922 patients), the primary end points occurred in 51 patients in the ximelagatran group and in 37 patients in the warfarin group (1.6% vs 1.2%, respectively, absolute difference 0.45%; 95% CI, −0.13%–1.03%; P<.001).[11] This study demonstrated ximelagatran to be noninferior to warfarin for the prevention of stroke and systemic embolism in relatively high-risk patients with AF.[11] Significantly more minor and major hemorrhages occurred in SPORTIF III in patients receiving warfarin than in those receiving ximelagatran (relative risk reduction [RRR] of ximelagatran, 14%; 95% CI, 4–22, P<.007).[10] Similarly, SPORTIF V demonstrated significantly fewer major and minor hemorrhagic events in the group receiving ximelagatran versus the group receiving warfarin (RRR, 21%; 95% CI, −14%–6.0% per year; P<.001).[9] Combined data from both studies showed a reduced relative risk of major hemorrhage, including intracranial hemorrhage, for ximelagatran versus warfarin (RRR 0.74; 95% CI, 0.57–0.97) and a reduced risk of minor and major hemorrhage (32.0% and 39.1% for the ximelagatran group and the warfarin group, respectively).[9,10,12] Elevations of ALT greater than 3 times the upper limit of normal were experienced by 6% of patients in the ximelagatran group compared with 0.8% of patients in the warfarin group (P<.001).[9] One patient died as a result of liver failure 20 days after cessation of ximelagatran use and was found to have hepatic necrosis on biopsy, while another patient's ALT was greater than 11 times the upper limit of normal and consequently suffered from a fatal gastrointestinal hemorrhage.[9]

Secondary Prevention of VTE

The treatment of high-density lipoproteins to reduce the incidence of vascular events (THRIVE) trial was a 6-month, randomized, double-blind, noninferiority study in 2490 patients with acute venous thromboembolism receiving oral ximelagatran 36 mg twice daily versus enoxaparin/warfarin. Recurrent VTE was found in 26 ximelagatran patients (2.1%) versus 24 enoxaparin/warfarin patients (2.0%) meeting prespecified noninferiority criteria (95% CI, −1.0%–1.3%). Rates of major bleeding were similar. ALT was greater than 3 times the upper limit of normal in 9.6% of ximelagatran patients versus 2.0% of warfarin patients.[13]

An extension of the THRIVE III study assessed prolonged prophylaxis with ximelagatran 24 mg twice daily versus placebo after 6 months of standard therapy or ximelagatran therapy. Symptomatic, recurrent venous thromboembolism occurred in 12 patients in the ximelagatran group versus 71 patients in the placebo group (hazard ratio [HR], 0.16; 95% CI, 0.09–0.30; P<.001).[14] Elevations of ALT greater than 3 times the upper limit of normal were seen in a larger portion of individuals assigned to the ximelagatran group versus the placebo group (6.4% vs 1.2%, respectively; P<.001).[14]

Treatment in Acute Coronary Syndrome

Efficacy and safety of oral direct thrombin inhibitor ximelagatran in patients with recent myocardial damage (ESTEEM) was a placebo-controlled, double-blind, phase 2 dose-guiding investigation of ximelagatran and aspirin (ASA) in individuals who had recent ST-elevation or non-ST elevation myocardial infarctions. The primary end point was the occurrence of death, nonfatal myocardial infarction, and severe recurrent ischemic events after a recent myocardial infarction.[15] All patients received ASA and either oral ximelagatran at varying doses (24 mg, 36 mg, 48 mg, or 60 mg twice daily) or placebo for a total of 6 months. At 6 months, ximelagatran was superior to placebo in reducing the cumulative risk of reaching an adverse outcome (16.3% for placebo vs 12.7% in the combined ximelagatran groups; HR, 0.76; 95% CI, 0.59–0.98, P = .036).[15] There was no difference in efficacy between the various doses of ximelagatran. An ALT level greater than 3 times the upper limit of normal was more frequent in the ximelagatran groups versus the placebo group (P<.0001),[15] and 4 patients developed an elevated serum bilirubin and ALT.[15]

Cessation of Ximelagatran Usage

Although ximelagatran was demonstrated to be as effective as traditional anticoagulants in the prevention and treatment of venous thrombosis and stroke prevention in AF, a signal of hepatotoxicity led the US Food and Drug Administration (FDA) agency to re-evaluate the benefits of long-term use of the drug. In the majority of patients who experienced transient elevations in liver enzymes, these levels returned to normal either spontaneously or with cessation of ximelagatran therapy.[2] Further investigations demonstrated that even regular monitoring of hepatic enzymes while on ximelagatran could not predict the severity of possible hepatic injury, and a 35-day study demonstrated that severe hepatic injury could result even after cessation of ximelagatran use.[16] Thus, after careful investigation and analysis of completed trials with ximelagatran, it was determined that the risks of the drug outweighed its benefits, and it was ultimately denied by the FDA in 2004.[12]

DABIGATRAN ETEXILATE

Dabigatran etexilate (PRADAXA, BIBR 1048) is the oral prodrug of dabigatran (BIBR 953), a low molecular weight molecule that acts as a specific, potent, and reversible direct thrombin inhibitor (DTI). Approved in Canada and Europe in 2008 for the prevention of VTE after elective total hip replacement and/or total knee replacement, dabigatran etexilate is not yet FDA-approved in the United States. The efficacy and safety of dabigatran etexilate compared with standard anticoagulant therapy is currently in phase 3 of development. The extensive RE-VOLUTION trial program supported by Boehringer Ingelheim includes multiple phase 3 trials that have focused on the use of dabigatran etexilate for primary VTE prevention after hip and knee surgeries, treatment of acute DVT and/or PE and their secondary prevention, prevention of stroke and systemic embolism in patients with nonvalvular AF, and secondary prevention of cardiac events in patients with acute coronary syndromes (ACS) (**Table 1**).

Studies of dabigatran etexilate in healthy volunteers have identified key clinical advantages of this drug, including a rapid conversion to its active form dabigatran, which has early peak plasma concentrations and a half-life between 12 and 17 hours, a predictable and consistent anticoagulant effect with low potential for drug-drug or drug-food interactions, and a lack of (or induction) metabolism by the cytochrome P450 enzymes. All of these characteristics allow dabigatran etexilate to be given as a fixed, once- or twice-daily dose without the need for coagulation monitoring.

Absorption and Metabolism of Dabigatran Etexilate and Dabigatran

Dabigatran is a 472 Da peptidomimetic that directly inhibits thrombin by binding to its active site via ionic interactions. It is a highly basic and hydrophilic compound and therefore has poor intestinal absorption after oral administration. To increase its bioavailability, the addition of a less basic, lipophilic side chain, N-hexyl carbamate ester, led to the development of a 628 Da, gastrointestinally absorbed double prodrug dabigatran etexilate. After oral administration, the prodrug is rapidly absorbed in the stomach and small intestine and converted to its active form, dabigatran, via 2 intermediate metabolites (BIBR 951 and BIBR 1087) through cleavage of the lipophilic

Table 1
Completed phase 3 trials comparing dabigatran etexilate with control therapy for prevention and treatment of thromboembolism

Study	Indication	Number of Patients	Dabigatran Etexilate Regimen	Comparator Regimen	1° Outcome Measure	1° Outcome Measure Results (%)	Serious Bleeding (%)
RE-MOBILIZE[31]	VTE prevention after TKR	2615	150 or 220 mg once-daily (starting with a half-dose 6–12 h postop) for 12–15 d	Enoxaparin 30 mg twice-daily starting postop for 12–15 d	Total VTE and all-cause mortality[32]	Dabigatran (150 mg), 33.7% Dabigatran (220 mg), 31.1% Enoxaparin, 25.3% Both dabigatran etexilate doses failed to show noninferiority to enoxaparin	Dabigatran (150 mg), 0.6% Dabigatran (220 mg), 0.6% Enoxaparin, 1.4%
RE-MODEL[32]	VTE prevention after TKR	2076	150 mg or 220 mg once-daily (starting with a half-dose 1–4 h postop) for 6–10 d	Enoxaparin 40 mg every day (starting the evening before surgery) for 6–10 d	Total VTE and all-cause mortality	Dabigatran (150 mg), 40.5% Dabigatran (220 mg), 36.4% Enoxaparin, 37.7% Both doses of dabigatran etexilate were noninferior to enoxaparin for VTE prevention	Dabigatran (150 mg), 1.3% Dabigatran (220 mg), 1.5% Enoxaparin, 1.3%
RE-NOVATE[33]	VTE prevention after THR	3494	150 or 220 mg once-daily (starting with a half-dose 1–4 h postop) for 28–35 d	Enoxaparin 40 mg once-daily preop for 28–35 d	Total VTE and all-cause mortality	Dabigatran (150 mg), 8.6% Dabigatran (220 mg), 6% Enoxaparin, 6.7% Both doses of dabigatran etexilate were noninferior to enoxaparin for VTE prevention	Dabigatran (150 mg), 1.3% Dabigatran (220 mg), 2% Enoxaparin, 1.6%
RE-COVER[34]	Treatment in acute VTE	2564	150 mg twice-daily (starting after 8–11 d of parenteral therapy) for 6 mo	Warfarin (dose adjusted for INR 2.0–3.0) after 8–11 d of initial parenteral anticoagulation	Recurrent VTE and related deaths	Dabigatran, 2.4% Warfarin, 2.1% Dabigatran etexilate is noninferior to warfarin in the prevention of recurrent or fatal VTE	Dabigatran, 16.1% Warfarin, 21.9%
RE-LY[36]	Prevention of stroke in nonvalvular atrial fibrillation	18,113	110 mg or 150 mg twice-daily for 2 y	Warfarin (dose adjusted for INR 2.0–3.0) for 2 y	Stroke and systemic embolism	Dabigatran (110 mg), 1.53%/y Dabigatran (150 mg), 1.11%/y Warfarin, 1.69%/y Both doses of dabigatran etexilate were noninferior to warfarin	Dabigatran (110 mg), 0.12%/y Dabigatran (150 mg), 0.10%/y Warfarin, 0.38%/y

Other phase 3 trials currently evaluating dabigatran etexilate include: RE-NOVATE II (VTE prevention post-THR); RE-COVER II (acute VTE treatment); RE-MEDY and RE-SONATE (secondary prevention of VTE); RE-LYABLE (stroke prevention in atrial fibrillation). A phase 2 trial currently evaluating dabigatran etexilate in the secondary prevention of cardiac events in ACS is RE-DEEM.

Abbreviations: Postop, postoperatively; Preop, preoperatively; THR, total hip replacement; TKR, total knee replacement; VTE (venous thromboembolism) includes deep vein thrombosis and pulmonary embolism.

ester moiety by rapidly acting serine esterase-catalyzed hydrolysis. The advantage of this ethyl ester-structured prodrug compared with other DTIs with hydroxylamine-structured prodrugs, such as ximelagatran, is that the P450 (CYP) isoenzymes or other oxidoreductases are not significantly involved in the proteolytic reactions that convert dabigatran etexilate to dabigatran. Also, in vitro studies reveal that dabigatran does not inhibit the cytochrome P450 enzymes.[17] Therefore, the potential for drug-drug interactions is low.

The bioavailability of dabigatran after oral absorption is low (6%–7%) and is independent of the dose of the prodrug.[17] The linear relationship between the prodrug dose and plasma concentrations of dabigatran excludes saturable first-pass elimination as the cause for low bioavailability.[18] Dose-escalation studies have shown that dabigatran plasma concentrations increase in a dose-proportional manner[18] and therefore, high doses of dabigatran etexilate are necessary to achieve adequate plasma concentrations. The absorption and metabolism of dabigatran etexilate is also dependent on an acidic microenvironment. The original tablet form used in the Boehringer Ingelheim Study in thrombosis (BISTRO) 1a trial resulted in low plasma concentrations of dabigatran after the first dose in 20% of the patients undergoing total hip replacement surgery, causing a high interindividual variability in the pharmacokinetic parameters.[19] Therefore, a new capsule formulation was developed, which contains multiple small pellets containing a tartaric acid core and coated with dabigatran etexilate.[18] Slight variations in intrinsic gastric pH have not significantly affected the extent of absorption of dabigatran etexilate. As a result of the improved dissolving characteristics, earlier postoperative administration of dabigatran etexilate has been possible, and an immediate onset of absorption and peak plasma concentrations at 6 hours after administration has been observed.[20]

After absorption of dabigatran etexilate, bioconversion to dabigatran occurs in enterocytes, hepatocytes, and portal vein. Glucuronic acid is conjugated with 20% of dabigatran to yield pharmacologically activated glucuronide conjugates that have almost exact properties as free, unconjugated dabigatran, and therefore have no impact on the efficacy of dabigatran.[17] Once metabolized to dabigatran, the prodrug and its intermediate metabolites, BIBR 951 and BIBR 1087, are trace detectable in the plasma of healthy subjects.[21] The absorption and metabolism of dabigatran etexilate has also been tested in patients with hepatic impairment. In patients with moderate hepatic impairment (Child-Pugh Category B), the bioconversion rate from dabigatran etexilate to its active form via the intermediate BIBR 1087 was slightly slower than that in matched healthy control subjects. The area under the plasma concentration-time curves (AUCs) for dabigatran etexilate and its intermediates BIBR 1087 and BIBR 951 relative to the AUC of dabigatran in plasma were 1.8%, 5.9%, and 0.3%, respectively, compared with AUCs of less than 0.4% in the healthy control group.[22]

Studies using radiolabeled (^{14}C) oral dabigatran etexilate and ^{14}C intravenous dabigatran show that dabigatran is the predominant compound in plasma, urine, and feces, and that more than 80% of systemically available dabigatran is renally excreted. The remainder undergoes conjugation with glucuronic acid to form acylglucuronides, which are excreted via the bile. Unchanged dabigatran accounts for approximately 77% of the intravenous dose of dabigatran and the remainder are glucuronide conjugates.[17] Dabigatran also has moderate tissue distribution, because the volume of distribution of dabigatran given by intravenous infusion is 60 to 70 L.[21]

Pharmacokinetic Characteristics of Dabigatran Etexilate and Dabigatran

The pharmacokinetic profile (PK) of dabigatran etexilate and dabigatran has been studied in healthy subjects, both young and old, and in patients undergoing hip arthroplasty or in those with AF at risk of cardioembolic events. Studies of healthy subjects not undergoing surgery reveal that dabigatran is well tolerated and that its time to peak plasma concentrations (C_{max}) is achieved within 1 to 3 hours following either single or multiple doses of oral administration of dabigatran etexilate, regardless of age or gender.[17,18,20,23] The onset of absorption is also immediate in healthy patients undergoing total hip replacement surgery; however, the rate and degree of absorption is slightly decreased in the first 24 hours postoperatively (C_{max} [75.8 ng/mL] is achieved at 6 hours). Despite these results found among surgical patients, the extent of absorption (mean $AUC_{0-24\ h}$) is acceptable and comparable to values obtained in healthy volunteers (962 and 904 ng/mL, respectively). The slower time progression to C_{max} with an unchanged AUC may help decrease the risk of bleeding in patients in the early postoperative period.[20] Studies in the orthopedic and elderly populations reveal that coadministration of pantoprazole reduces overall drug exposure by 20% to 25%, although this may not be clinically relevant.[20,24] Food prolongs the time to peak plasma dabigatran levels by 2 hours without effect on its extent of absorption (AUC).[20] In addition, the PK is not affected by the use of comedications, such as opioids,[20] diclofenac,[25] atorvastatin,[26] or digoxin.[24] However, a reduced dose of dabigatran etexilate is recommended when coadministered with amiodarone, because studies in patients taking amiodarone who underwent orthopedic procedures showed an increased C_{max} and AUC for dabigatran.[25]

Early clinical studies also reveal time- and dose-independent pharmacokinetics of dabigatran. There is a proportional and steady increase in the C_{max} and AUC with increasing single or multiple doses of dabigatran etexilate. After absorption, a rapid distribution phase occurs followed by a prolonged elimination time. The mean plasma terminal half-life of dabigatran in healthy young and elderly adults is 12 to 14 hours,[18,21,23] independent of dose, and accordingly, steady-state concentrations are attained in 3 days with multiple dosing and without evidence of significant accumulation.[23] Although 35% of dabigatran is bound to plasma proteins, it is unlikely that displacement interactions affect its pharmacokinetics or pharmacodynamics.[17]

Renal insufficiency is natural and common in the elderly, and age-related reduction in creatinine clearance (CL_{CR}) is associated with decreased elimination of dabigatran. Increased trough concentrations have been reported in patients with CL_{CR} less than 50 mL/min.[25] The bioavailability of dabigatran is 1.7 to 2.0 times greater in elderly subjects than in young healthy subjects of the same sex.[23] Also, the extent of exposure (AUC) to dabigatran is 2.7- and 6-fold greater with moderate (CL_{CR} 30–50 mL/min) or severe renal insufficiency (CL_{CR} 10–30 mL/min, respectively).[21] Therefore, dose reduction of dabigatran etexilate is appropriate in the elderly or patients with renal insufficiency (CL_{CR} <50 mL/min).[21,24] Gender-dependent differences in CR_{CL} with downstream differences in dabigatran exposure are also apparent (mean AUC ~3%–19% higher in elderly women) yet do not require modifications in dosing.[23] Although dabigatran is dialyzable, it is contraindicated in patients with severe renal impairment (CL_{CR} <30 mL/min).[21]

Pharmacodynamic Characteristics of Dabigatran Etexilate and Dabigatran

In vitro studies show that dabigatran rapidly and reversibly inhibits clot-bound and free thrombin in a concentration-dependent manner with an inhibition constant (K_i) of 4.5 nmol/L.[27] Its specificity is highly selective for thrombin over other serine proteases. In addition, dabigatran inhibits thrombin-activated human platelet aggregation with a half maximal inhibitory concentration (IC_{50}) value of 10 nmol/L.[27] Tissue factor–induced thrombin generation in human platelet-poor plasma is also inhibited by dabigatran in a concentration-dependent manner.[27]

Different clot-based assays have been used to assess the pharmacodynamic effects of dabigatran. The activated partial thromboplastin time (aPTT) assay measures the time to thrombin generation and clot formation via the intrinsic pathway, which involves fibrinogen and factors II, V, X, VIII, IX, XI, and XII, whereas the PT assay represents the clotting time in the extrinsic pathway involving fibrinogen and factors II, V, X, and VII. The thrombin time (TT) and ecarin clotting time (ECT) tests also measure the time to clot formation by directly measuring the activity of thrombin and the inhibitory activity of the DTI. In the latter test ecarin is used, which converts prothrombin into its intermediate meixothrombin, another substrate that is inhibited by dabigatran.[18] It has been shown that prolongation of clotting times (aPTT, PT, TT, ECT) occurs in parallel with increasing concentrations of dabigatran, and that peak clotting times coincide with the C_{max} of dabigatran (2 hours after oral administration). This observation suggests that the effects of dabigatran on thrombin inhibition are rapid and without a time delay. Similarly, at the time of the first half-life (12 hours after oral administration) of dabigatran, the prolongation of blood coagulation returned to 50% of the maximum effect.

TT and ECT both exhibit a linear dose-response relationship with therapeutic concentrations of dabigatran; however, because 50-fold prolongations of the TT have been reported, the TT coagulation test may prove to be too sensitive in the clinically relevant plasma concentration range. The ECT assay may be a more useful test for measuring thrombin inhibition and has been reported as having adequate sensitivity and precision with predictable and reproducible results.[24] Prolongation of the aPTT also occurs with increasing plasma concentrations of dabigatran but in a nonlinear manner. A plateau in aPTT prolongation is noted at high dabigatran concentrations (>400 ng/mL). These observations suggest that the aPTT coagulation assay may not be acceptable as a precise measurement of anticoagulation, particularly at high doses of dabigatran. Prothrombin time is not affected by dabigatran at clinically relevant plasma concentrations. The intersubject variability of aPTT, PT, TT, and ECT is low, with a coefficient of variation ranging from 6% to 11%.[28] Given the predictable pharmacokinetics and pharmacodynamics of dabigatran and its lack of drug-drug interactions, careful coagulation monitoring is not needed.

Prevention of Venous Thromboembolism After Orthopedic Surgery

The preclinical and early-phase clinical trials established predictable pharmacokinetic and pharmacodynamic profiles for dabigatran. Two phase 2 clinical trials, involving more than 2000 patients, were conducted to examine the safe therapeutic range of dabigatran etexilate and its optimal dosing regimens for prevention of venous thromboembolism following orthopedic surgery. In both studies, the primary efficacy outcome was the rate of thromboembolic events during the treatment period, while the primary safety outcome was the incidence of major bleeding.[19,29]

BISTRO trials consisted of 2 large studies that investigated the dose-response relationships and the safety and efficacy of dabigatran etexilate in VTE prevention for patients undergoing total elective hip and knee replacement surgery. BISTRO 1a was an open-label, multicenter dose-escalation study of dabigatran etexilate in 314 patients undergoing hip replacement surgery. Patients received 1 of 9 doses (12.5, 25, 50, 100, 150, 200, and 300 mg twice daily or 150 vs 300 mg once daily) of the tablet formulation of dabigatran etexilate beginning 4 to 8 hours after surgery for total treatment duration of 6 to 10 days.[19]

The BISTRO 1a study showed a relatively low incidence of DVT rates across all doses of dabigatran etexilate, with an overall rate of 12.4%. Pharmacokinetic and pharmacodynamic parameters increased proportionally with dose. The highest rates of DVT (20.8%) were found in the group receiving 12.5 mg twice daily as opposed to 6.1% in the 300 mg once-daily group. Regarding safety, an increased incidence of bleeding events was noted with higher doses of dabigatran etexilate. Although no major bleeding episodes were observed at any of the doses studied, the dose-escalation was terminated at 300 mg twice daily because 2 patients who received this dose experienced bleeding from multiple sites. This study concluded that a therapeutic window between 12 mg once daily and 300 mg twice daily was considered acceptable for its efficacy and safety.[19]

Because the BISTRO 1a study revealed low plasma concentrations of dabigatran after the first dose of the tablet formulation in 20% of patients, BISTRO 1b was conducted to evaluate the efficacy of the capsule formulation of dabigatran etexilate. The data showed that absorption of the first postoperative dose (1–3 hours after surgery) occurred slowly compared with healthy controls. Peak plasma concentrations were achieved in 6 hours following administration; however, on subsequent days the absorption of dabigatran was rapid (time to C_{max} = 2 hours). This delay in absorption on the first postoperative day may represent a "safety net" for these patients given their high risk of bleeding.[20] Thus, this PK justified the use of the capsule form and early dosing regimen to evaluate dabigatran etexilate on clinical outcomes in the BISTRO II study.

BISTRO II trial was a large, multicenter, parallel-group, randomized double-blind study whose primary objectives were to further evaluate the efficacy and safety of the dose-response relationship of dabigatran etexilate for VTE prevention in patients undergoing hip and knee replacement surgery, as well as to compare these outcomes against the current standard therapy, low molecular weight heparin (enoxaparin). Patients were randomized to receive doses of dabigatran etexilate of 50, 150, or 225 mg twice daily, or 300 mg once daily, versus enoxaparin 40 mg once daily. Results of the study again demonstrated a dose-dependent decrease in total VTE with increasing doses of dabigatran etexilate. Also, the incidence of major VTE (proximal DVT and/or PE) was lower in groups with any dose of dabigatran etexilate (1.7%–5.0%) than with enoxaparin (5.6%). Investigators concluded that a total daily dose of 100 to 300 mg of dabigatran etexilate appeared to be as effective as 40 mg of enoxaparin once daily; however, larger studies were recommended to assess the risk of bleeding. An equally important finding was the association between early administration of dabigatran etexilate (1–4 hours postoperative) and a reduced risk of DVT. Further pharmacokinetic and pharmacodynamic studies on patients enrolled in BISTRO II supported a dosing regimen for phase 3 trials, consisting of once-daily doses of 150 mg or 220 mg, with half doses of 75 mg and 110 mg given on the day of surgery.[29]

Pooled analysis of the results from the completed RE-MOBLIZE, RE-MODEL, and RE-NOVATE phase 3 trials, which involved a combined total of 8210 patients, determined that dabigatran etexilate is as efficacious and safe as enoxaparin in the prevention of VTE after hip or knee arthroplasty.[30] Two different doses of dabigatran etexilate, 150 mg or 220 mg once daily with half doses, 75 mg or 110 mg, on the first day were examined in all 3 trials. The lower dose of dabigatran etexilate was reserved for patients with a higher risk of bleeding, such as in those with reduced creatinine clearance or the elderly patients. The North American approved regimen of enoxaparin, 30 mg twice daily beginning 12 to 24 hours after surgery, was the comparator in the RE-MOBILIZE[31] trial, whereas the European enoxaparin regimen of 40 mg daily starting 12 hours before surgery was used as the comparator in RE-MODEL[32] and RE-NOVATE.[33] It is also noteworthy that the first dose of dabigatran etexilate was administered 6 to 12 hours after surgery in RE-MOBLIZE, whereas in RE-MODEL and RE-NOVATE prophylaxis began 1 to 4 hours postoperatively.

Results from RE-MOBILIZE failed to show noninferiority of dabigatran to enoxaparin. The primary end point, total VTE and all-cause mortality rates, were significantly higher in the dabigatran 220 mg (31.1%; $P = .02$) and 150 mg (33.7%; $P<.001$) groups compared with enoxaparin (25.3%). Rates of major bleeding were not significantly different between dabigatran groups and the enoxaparin group. The failure to achieve noninferiority is likely secondary to the delay in the administration of dabigatran etexilate after surgery as well as the higher dosing of enoxaparin.[31]

RE-MODEL and RE-NOVATE, both performed in the European Union and other non–North American countries, found both doses of dabigatran noninferior to enoxaparin. Rates of total VTE and all-cause mortality were 36.4% ($P<.0003$) and 40.5% ($P<.017$) for doses of 220 mg and 150 mg, respectively, versus 37.7% for enoxaparin in RE-MODEL.[32] Similar findings were observed in RE-NOVATE (6.0% [$P<.0001$], 8.6% [$P<.0001$], and 6.7% in dabigatran 220 mg, 150 mg, and enoxaparin 40 mg daily, respectively).[33] In both studies, rates of major bleeding events were similar across all treatment groups. Administration of dabigatran etexilate beginning 1 to 4 hours postoperatively in both trials with resultant improved outcomes support early administration of thromboprophylaxis. Data from these 2 trials led to the approval of dabigatran etexilate for the primary prevention of VTE after total knee or hip replacement in the European Union and Canada. A fourth phase 3 trial, RE-NOVATE II, is currently ongoing in North America with a goal to evaluate the efficacy of dabigatran 220 mg once daily versus enoxaparin 40 mg once daily over a course of 28 to 35 days for VTE prevention post hip replacement surgery.

Pooled results from the 3 trials revealed no statistically significant difference between both doses of dabigatran etexilate versus the comparator enoxaparin for the primary end point of total VTE and all-cause mortality (RR 1.06, 95% CI 0.94–1.18), as well as the secondary end point of major VTE or VTE-related death (RR 0.92, 95% CI 0.66–1.29). Similarly, a lack of a statistically significant difference in major bleeding events between dabigatran etexilate 220 mg and 150 mg treatment groups (1.4% and 1.1%, respectively) versus enoxaparin (1.4%) was observed. Further post hoc pooled analysis in elderly patients (>75 years) recommended a 150 mg daily dose of dabigatran etexilate for prevention of VTE. This dose may extend to other patients at higher risk of bleeding, such as those taking amiodarone or verapamil, or with a creatinine clearance less than 50 mL/min.[30]

SECONDARY PREVENTION OF VENOUS THROMBOEMBOLISM

The RE-COVER trial was another large, randomized, noninferiority trial that demonstrated dabigatran etexilate to have a similar efficacy and safety profile as warfarin in the treatment of acute symptomatic venous thromboembolism. Patients (n = 2539) with acute, symptomatic, objectively verified proximal DVT of the legs or PE were randomized to receive 6 months of either oral dabigatran etexilate 150 mg twice daily or warfarin (adjusted for INR 2–3) after initial parenteral anticoagulation therapy (median = 9 days). The primary end point was either recurrent venous thromboembolism or fatal PE during the treatment period that occurred in 2.4% of patients treated with dabigatran compared with 2.1% of patients receiving warfarin. Fatal bleeding occurred in 1 patient in each treatment arm, and intracranial bleeding was absent in the dabigatran group while being present in 3 patients from the warfarin arm. An HR of 1.10 (95% CI, 0.65–1.84) for dabigatran established its noninferiority to warfarin. Rates of major bleeding with dabigatran were similar to warfarin (1.6% vs 1.9%, respectively); however, a significant decrease in any bleeding events was observed for dabigatran when compared with warfarin (16.1% vs 21.9%; HR 0.71 [95% CI,

0.59–0.85; *P*<.001]).[34] A limitation of this study was that dabigatran was first administered to patients only after initial parenteral anticoagulation. Earlier studies have repeatedly shown dabigatran to have a rapid onset of effect yet monotherapy with dabigatran was not evaluated in this trial.

A second trial comparing dabigatran etexilate to warfarin in the treatment of acute VTE is underway (RE-COVER II). Two trials (RE-MEDY and RE-SONATE) are currently ongoing to evaluate dabigatran etexilate against warfarin in the long-term secondary prevention of venous thromboembolism.

Stroke Prevention in AF

The Prevention of Embolic and ThROmbotic events in patients with persistent non-valvular atrial fibrillation (PETRO) was a double-blind, dose-escalating phase 2 trial that evaluated the efficacy of dabigatran in the prevention of thromboembolic events.[35] PETRO-Ex was a long-term, open-label extension phase 2 trial for those taking dabigatran in PETRO. The primary outcome was the frequency of bleeding events. Patients (n = 502) were randomized to receive dabigatran etexilate (50, 150, or 300 mg twice daily) with or without aspirin (81 or 325 mg daily) and compared with warfarin alone (adjusted to INR = 2–3) for 12 weeks. Excessive bleeding was identified in those groups taking aspirin (81 or 325 mg) with 300 mg dabigatran etexilate, resulting in termination of the allowable use of aspirin within the study. A dose-dependent increase in bleeding was found in dabigatran etexilate 300 mg and 150 mg groups compared with the 50 mg groups (*P* = .0002, *P* = .01, respectively). Thromboembolic events were observed with the 50 mg dabigatran dose groups (2 of 107, 2%), and a dose of 150 mg twice daily was concluded to be as effective as the higher dose and warfarin. From the results of this study, dabigatran etexilate doses of 200 to 300 mg daily for phase 3 testing in the prevention of thromboembolic events in patients with AF was recommended.[35]

Results from the randomized evaluation of long-term anticoagulation therapy (RE-LY) phase 3 trial have been recently published. A large, prospective, randomized, open, blinded end point, noninferiority trial, RE-LY involved 18,113 patients with AF and at least one additional risk factor for stroke (CHADS$_2$ score ≥1). The efficacy and safety of 2 blinded doses of dabigatran etexilate (150 and 110 mg twice a day) versus open-label warfarin (adjusted for target INR 2–3) in the prevention of stroke (including hemorrhagic stroke) or systemic embolism during a follow-up period of 2 years was compared. RE-LY showed that the rate (percent per year) of the primary outcome (stroke or systemic embolism) was significantly lower with dabigatran etexilate 150 mg twice daily (1.11%) and noninferior with 110 mg twice daily (1.53%) compared with warfarin (1.69%). A dabigatran etexilate dose of 150 mg twice a day (0.92%) was also superior to warfarin (1.20%) in preventing nonhemorrhagic stroke; however, dabigatran etexilate at a dose of 110 mg twice a day was not (1.34%). The rates of hemorrhagic stroke were significantly lower with 150 mg (0.10%, *P*<.001) and 110 mg (0.12%, *P*<.001) twice-daily doses of dabigatran etexilate versus warfarin (0.38%). The rate of major bleeding was significantly higher in the group receiving warfarin (3.36%) compared with those receiving the lower dose of dabigatran (2.71% for 110 mg twice a day) and was noninferior to those receiving the higher dose (3.11% for 150 mg twice a day). The study concluded that when compared with adjusted-dose warfarin, a dabigatran etexilate dose of 110 mg twice daily was associated with a similar rate of stroke but less risk of major bleeding, whereas a dose of 150 mg twice daily prevented more strokes but had a similar rate of major hemorrhage.[36] A long-term study, RELY-ABLE, is currently underway to evaluate the safety profile of dabigatran in these patients. These findings also suggest the potential ability to appropriately choose the dose of dabigatran depending on the patient's risk profile for stroke and bleeding.

Adverse effects

Like all other anticoagulants, bleeding is the major complication. However, phase 2 and phase 3 studies have shown that the risk of bleeding with dabigatran etexilate is equivalent to or less then that with warfarin. These studies also showed that unlike ximelagatran, dabigatran is not associated with hepatic toxicity. However, the rate of myocardial infarctions was higher with both doses of dabigatran than with warfarin in RE-LY, whereas in RE-COVER, the number of myocardial infarcts was similar between the 2 treatment groups. The most common adverse side effect of dabigatran etexilate reported in these studies was dyspepsia.

OTHER ORAL IIA INHIBITORS

In addition to dabigatran etexilate, other novel DTIs are currently being evaluated in phase 1, 2, and 3 studies for the prevention of venous thromboembolism. After discontinuing ximelagatran, AstraZeneca produced AZD0837, a prodrug that is rapidly converted to its active form, H067637, via the intermediate H069927, and which has been reported to have superior pharmacologic properties compared with ximelagatran without its associated toxicities. It has an oral bioavailability of 22% to 55% and a time to C_{max} of 0.7 to 1.5 hours after oral administration. The half-life of H067637 is 9 hours after a single dose; however, the development of an extended release formulation allows once-daily administration.[37] Phase 2 studies have investigated the efficacy and safety of AZD0837 in the prevention of systemic embolism and stroke in patients with AF. The phase 2 trial was a randomized, parallel, dose-guiding study that compared AZD0837 doses of 150 mg twice a day or 350 mg twice a day to warfarin (adjusted for goal INR 2–3). The results showed that a dose of AZD0837 150 mg twice a day had a similar efficacy and tolerability profile as warfarin.[37] Gastrointestinal side effects were noted at increasing doses of AZD0837. AZD0837 has now entered a large phase 3 warfarin-controlled trial to determine its efficacy and safety for stroke prevention in AF.

SB-424323 (Odiparcil) is an oral β-D-xyloside that indirectly inhibits thrombin via heparin cofactor II.[38] Its efficacy and safety was evaluated in the phase 2a, randomized, placebo-controlled study, ThromboEMbolism Prevention Efficacy and Safety Trial (TEMPEST), which involved 225 patients undergoing total hip replacement surgery. When compared against placebo, odiparcil doses of 125 mg or 500 mg twice daily significantly reduced the rate of VTE compared with placebo (6.5% and 3.9%, respectively vs 15.5%).[39] A dose-ranging phase 2b trial (TOPVENT) is currently ongoing to compare odiparcil to warfarin in the prevention of venous thromboembolism in patients undergoing total knee replacement surgery.[39]

TGN-167 (TRI-50c-04) is another novel oral DTI undergoing evaluation for the prevention of arterial and venous thrombosis. Pharmacokinetic studies show it to have a predictable and stable PK with a marked increase in thrombin clotting time and minimal effects on aPTT. In a double-blind, phase 1 dose-escalating study involving 20 healthy male volunteers, TGN-167 was found to be well tolerated and without significant adverse events. In vitro effective anticoagulant activity was found in all of the subjects, given a dose of 600 mg.[40] Phase 2 studies for TGN-167 are planned. Also being developed is a controlled-release formulation of TGN-167. Other potential DTIs in early phase clinical studies include SSR182289A (Sanofi-Synthelabo), aptamer ARC-183 (Archemix-Nuvelo), LB-30870 (LG Life Sciences), GW473178 (GlaxoSmithKline), MCC-977 (Mitsubishi Pharma), and TGN-255 (Trigen Holdings).[41]

SUMMARY

Oral IIa inhibitors represent a new era of anticoagulation in the prevention and treatment of venous and arterial thromboembolism. At present, dabigatran etexilate is the most promising of the oral DTIs, offering more advantages over the traditional anticoagulants such as warfarin and even heparin. It inhibits circulating and clot-bound thrombin, and has a predictable and reliable pharmacokinetic and pharmacodynamic profile. Its lack of interaction with cytochrome P450 enzymes or with other food and drugs, rapid onset of action, excellent safety profile, lack of need for routine monitoring, broad therapeutic window, and fixed-dose administration make this a competitive anticoagulant.

However, more research is required to evaluate the safety of DTIs when used in conjunction with antiplatelet medications for the prevention and treatment of arterial thromboses. Also, the potential for long-term nonhematologic side effects needs to be addressed. Whether DTIs offer other nonhematologic advantages, such as those seen with heparin-based agents (ie, antitumor, anti-inflammatory, and immunoregulatory effects), remain to be determined. Lastly, head-to-head trials comparing oral FXa inhibitors to DTIs for the same indications need to be performed. Regardless, the new oral DTIs under investigation show promise in addressing the unmet needs of existing anticoagulants and give hope for a bright future for a new class of therapies aimed at the prevention and treatment of thromboembolic diseases.

REFERENCES

1. Gustafsson D, Nystrom J, Carlsson S, et al. The direct thrombin inhibitor melagatran and its oral prodrug H 376/95: intestinal absorption properties, biochemical and pharmacodynamic effects. Thromb Res 2001;101(3):171–81.
2. Bergsrud EA, Gandhi PJ. A review of the clinical uses of ximelagatran in thrombosis syndromes. J Thromb Thrombolysis 2003;16(3):175–88.
3. Crowther MA, Weitz JI. Ximelagatran: the first oral direct thrombin inhibitor. Expert Opin Investig Drugs 2004;13(4):403–13.
4. Eriksson BI, Agnelli G, Cohen AT, et al. Direct thrombin inhibitor melagatran followed by oral ximelagatran in comparison with enoxaparin for prevention of venous thromboembolism after total hip or knee replacement. Thromb Haemost 2003;89(2):288–96.
5. Eriksson BI, Agnelli G, Cohen AT, et al. The direct thrombin inhibitor melagatran followed by oral ximelagatran compared with enoxaparin for the prevention of venous thromboembolism after total hip or knee replacement: the EXPRESS study. J Thromb Haemost 2003;1(12):2490–6.
6. Colwell CW Jr, Berkowitz SD, Davidson BL, et al. Comparison of ximelagatran, an oral direct thrombin inhibitor, with enoxaparin for the prevention of venous thromboembolism following total hip replacement. A randomized, double-blind study. J Thromb Haemost 2003;1(10):2119–30.
7. Francis CW, Berkowitz SD, Comp PC, et al. Comparison of ximelagatran with warfarin for the prevention of venous thromboembolism after total knee replacement. N Engl J Med 2003;349(18):1703–12.
8. Colwell CW Jr, Berkowitz SD, Lieberman JR, et al. Oral direct thrombin inhibitor ximelagatran compared with warfarin for the prevention of venous thromboembolism after total knee arthroplasty. J Bone Joint Surg Am 2005;87(10):2169–77.
9. Halperin JL. Ximelagatran compared with warfarin for prevention of thromboembolism in patients with nonvalvular atrial fibrillation: Rationale, objectives, and

design of a pair of clinical studies and baseline patient characteristics (SPORTIF III and V). Am Heart J 2003;146(3):431–8.

10. Olsson SB. Stroke prevention with the oral direct thrombin inhibitor ximelagatran compared with warfarin in patients with non-valvular atrial fibrillation (SPORTIF III): randomised controlled trial. Lancet 2003;362(9397):1691–8.

11. Albers GW, Diener HC, Frison L, et al. Ximelagatran vs warfarin for stroke prevention in patients with nonvalvular atrial fibrillation: a randomized trial. JAMA 2005; 293(6):690–8.

12. O'Brien CL, Gage BF. Costs and effectiveness of ximelagatran for stroke prophylaxis in chronic atrial fibrillation. JAMA 2005;293(6):699–706.

13. Fiessinger JN, Huisman MV, Davidson BL, et al. Ximelagatran vs low-molecular-weight heparin and warfarin for the treatment of deep vein thrombosis: a randomized trial. JAMA 2005;293(6):681–9.

14. Schulman S, Wahlander K, Lundstrom T, et al. Secondary prevention of venous thromboembolism with the oral direct thrombin inhibitor ximelagatran. N Engl J Med 2003;349(18):1713–21.

15. Wallentin L, Wilcox RG, Weaver WD, et al. Oral ximelagatran for secondary prophylaxis after myocardial infarction: the ESTEEM randomised controlled trial. Lancet 2003;362(9386):789–97.

16. Keisu M, Andersson TB. Drug-induced liver injury in humans: the case of ximelagatran. Handb Exp Pharmacol 2010;196:407–18.

17. Blech S, Ebner T, Ludwig-Schwellinger E, et al. The metabolism and disposition of the oral direct thrombin inhibitor, dabigatran, in humans. Drug Metab Dispos 2008;36(2):386–99.

18. Stangier J, Rathgen K, Stahle H, et al. The pharmacokinetics, pharmacodynamics and tolerability of dabigatran etexilate, a new oral direct thrombin inhibitor, in healthy male subjects. Br J Clin Pharmacol 2007;64(3):292–303.

19. Eriksson BI, Dahl OE, Ahnfelt L, et al. Dose escalating safety study of a new oral direct thrombin inhibitor, dabigatran etexilate, in patients undergoing total hip replacement: BISTRO I. J Thromb Haemost 2004;2(9):1573–80.

20. Stangier J, Eriksson BI, Dahl OE, et al. Pharmacokinetic profile of the oral direct thrombin inhibitor dabigatran etexilate in healthy volunteers and patients undergoing total hip replacement. J Clin Pharmacol 2005;45(5):555–63.

21. Eriksson BI, Quinlan DJ, Weitz JI. Comparative pharmacodynamics and pharmacokinetics of oral direct thrombin and factor xa inhibitors in development. Clin Pharmacokinet 2009;48(1):1–22.

22. Stangier J, Stahle H, Rathgen K, et al. Pharmacokinetics and pharmacodynamics of dabigatran etexilate, an oral direct thrombin inhibitor, are not affected by moderate hepatic impairment. J Clin Pharmacol 2008;48(12):1411–9.

23. Stangier J, Stahle H, Rathgen K, et al. Pharmacokinetics and pharmacodynamics of the direct oral thrombin inhibitor dabigatran in healthy elderly subjects. Clin Pharmacokinet 2008;47(1):47–59.

24. Stangier J. Clinical pharmacokinetics and pharmacodynamics of the oral direct thrombin inhibitor dabigatran etexilate. Clin Pharmacokinet 2008;47(5): 285–95.

25. Stangier J, Clemens A. Pharmacology, pharmacokinetics, and pharmacodynamics of dabigatran etexilate, an oral direct thrombin inhibitor. Clin Appl Thromb Hemost 2009. [Epub ahead of print].

26. Stangier J, Rathgen K, Stahle H, et al. Coadministration of dabigatran etexilate and atorvastatin: assessment of potential impact on pharmacokinetics and pharmacodynamics. Am J Cardiovasc Drugs 2009;9(1):59–68.

27. Wienen W, Stassen JM, Priepke H, et al. In vitro profile and ex-vivo anticoagulant activity of the direct thrombin inhibitor dabigatran and its orally active prodrug, dabigatran etexilate. Thromb Haemost 2007;98(1):155–62.

28. Sorbera L, Bozzo J, Castaner J. Dabigatran/dabigatran etexilate. Drugs Future 2005;30(9):877–85.

29. Eriksson BI, Dahl OE, Buller HR, et al. A new oral direct thrombin inhibitor, dabigatran etexilate, compared with enoxaparin for prevention of thromboembolic events following total hip or knee replacement: the BISTRO II randomized trial. J Thromb Haemost 2005;3(1):103–11.

30. Wolowacz SE, Roskell NS, Plumb JM, et al. Efficacy and safety of dabigatran etexilate for the prevention of venous thromboembolism following total hip or knee arthroplasty. A meta-analysis. Thromb Haemost 2009;101(1):77–85.

31. Ginsberg JS, Davidson BL, Comp PC, et al. Oral thrombin inhibitor dabigatran etexilate vs North American enoxaparin regimen for prevention of venous thromboembolism after knee arthroplasty surgery. J Arthroplasty 2009;24(1):1–9.

32. Eriksson BI, Dahl OE, Rosencher N, et al. Oral dabigatran etexilate vs. subcutaneous enoxaparin for the prevention of venous thromboembolism after total knee replacement: the RE-MODEL randomized trial. J Thromb Haemost 2007;5(11):2178–85.

33. Eriksson BI, Dahl OE, Rosencher N, et al. Dabigatran etexilate versus enoxaparin for prevention of venous thromboembolism after total hip replacement: a randomised, double-blind, non-inferiority trial. Lancet 2007;370(9591):949–56.

34. Schulman S, Kearon C, Kakkar AK, et al. Dabigatran versus warfarin in the treatment of acute venous thromboembolism. N Engl J Med 2009;361(24):2342–52.

35. Ezekowitz MD, Reilly PA, Nehmiz G, et al. Dabigatran with or without concomitant aspirin compared with warfarin alone in patients with nonvalvular atrial fibrillation (PETRO Study). Am J Cardiol 2007;100(9):1419–26.

36. Connolly SJ, Ezekowitz MD, Yusuf S, et al. Dabigatran versus warfarin in patients with atrial fibrillation. N Engl J Med 2009;361(12):1139–51.

37. Olsson SB, Rasmussen LH, Tveit A, et al. Safety and tolerability of an immediate-release formulation of the oral direct thrombin inhibitor AZD0837 in the prevention of stroke and systemic embolism in patients with atrial fibrillation. Thromb Haemost 2010;103:604–12.

38. Upreti VV, Khurana M, Cox DS, et al. Determination of endogenous glycosaminoglycans derived disaccharides in human plasma by HPLC: validation and application in a clinical study. J Chromatogr B Analyt Technol Biomed Life Sci 2006;831(1–2):156–62.

39. Eriksson BI, Quinlan DJ. Oral anticoagulants in development: focus on thromboprophylaxis in patients undergoing orthopaedic surgery. Drugs 2006;66(11):1411–29.

40. Spyropoulos AC. Investigational treatments of venous thromboembolism. Expert Opin Investig Drugs 2007;16(4):431–40.

41. Schwienhorst A. Direct thrombin inhibitors—a survey of recent developments. Cell Mol Life Sci 2006;63(23):2773–91.

Agents for the Treatment of Heparin-Induced Thrombocytopenia

Theodore E. Warkentin, MD[a,b,c,d],*

KEYWORDS

- Heparin-induced thrombocytopenia • Coumarin necrosis
- Hirudin • Argatroban • Danaparoid • Fondaparinux

Heparin-induced thrombocytopenia (HIT) is an adverse drug reaction caused by platelet-activating immunoglobulin G (IgG) antibodies that recognize complexes of platelet factor 4 (PF4) bound to heparin. HIT is highly prothrombotic: at least 50% of affected patients develop thrombosis involving veins, arteries, or even the microcirculation.[1,2]

Even among patients without clinically evident thrombosis ("isolated HIT"), consensus conference guidelines[3,4] recommend therapy with a nonheparin anticoagulant, provided that the diagnosis of HIT is confirmed or strongly suspected on clinical grounds; this is because simple discontinuation of heparin, or substitution of heparin with warfarin, is associated with a subsequent risk for symptomatic thrombosis of between 35% and 50%, and for sudden fatal thrombosis of approximately 5%.[1,5]

A diagnosis of HIT usually signifies—rightly or wrongly—that all heparin preparations, including unfractionated heparin (UFH) and low-molecular-weight heparin

---

Studies cited[1,6,12–16,18,19,22,25,32–36,40,41,43,44,46–49,56,59,61,62,74,75] were supported by the Heart and Stroke Foundation of Ontario (operating grants #A2449, #T2967, B3763, #T4502, T#5207, and T#6157).

Disclosure: T.E.W. discloses consultancy, research support, and/or speaking fees from companies (Canyon Pharmaceutical, GTI Inc, GlaxoSmithKline, Organon Inc, Sanofi-Aventis) whose products are discussed in this article.

[a] Department of Pathology and Molecular Medicine, Michael G. DeGroote School of Medicine, McMaster University, Hamilton, ON, Canada
[b] Department of Medicine, Michael G. DeGroote School of Medicine, McMaster University, Hamilton, ON, Canada
[c] Transfusion Medicine, Hamilton Regional Laboratory Medicine Program, Hamilton, ON, Canada
[d] Service of Clinical Hematology, Hamilton Health Sciences, Hamilton General Hospital, Hamilton, ON, Canada
* Hamilton Regional Laboratory Medicine Program, Hamilton Health Sciences, Hamilton General Hospital, Room 1-180A, 237 Barton Street East, Hamilton, ON L8L 2X2, Canada.
E-mail address: twarken@mcmaster.ca

Hematol Oncol Clin N Am 24 (2010) 755–775
doi:10.1016/j.hoc.2010.05.009
0889-8588/10/$ – see front matter

hemonc.theclinics.com

(LMWH), are contraindicated. (Whether this is true or not is uncertain; in the author's experience, severe complications occur at least as often *after* stopping heparin as when its use is continued.) However, there is little doubt that initiating or maintaining warfarin therapy during HIT-associated hypercoagulability is an important risk factor for microvascular thrombosis, including the syndrome of warfarin-associated venous limb gangrene.[6] Thus, the "contraindication" status of UFH, LMWH, and warfarin during acute HIT necessarily means that novel anticoagulants have attained a prominent role in the management of HIT.

Three nonheparin anticoagulants—recombinant hirudin (r-hirudin), argatroban, and danaparoid—are approved in many jurisdictions for treatment of HIT[7–9] (an exception: danaparoid is neither approved for HIT nor available in the United States). Two other anticoagulants—fondaparinux and bivalirudin—are approved for non-HIT indications, but are used "off-label" for HIT.[10,11] These 5 anticoagulants can be divided into 2 groups: (1) long-acting, antithrombin 3 (AT3)-dependent, factor Xa inhibiting oligosaccharides (danaparoid, fondaparinux), and (2) short-acting, AT3-independent (ie, direct), thrombin inhibiting agents (r-hirudin, bivalirudin, argatroban), known as direct thrombin inhibitors (DTIs). The thesis of this review is that *for most patients with HIT the indirect factor Xa–inhibiting agents have the greatest therapeutic efficacy.*

HIT: A CLINICAL-PATHOLOGIC SYNDROME

HIT can be defined as any clinical event (or events) best explained by platelet-activating anti-PF4/heparin antibodies ("HIT antibodies," or HIT-Abs) in a patient who is receiving, or who has recently received, heparin.[12] Thrombocytopenia is the most common event in HIT, and is observed in at least 90% to 95% of patients, depending on how thrombocytopenia is defined.

HIT is a clinical-pathologic syndrome: thus, the diagnosis requires (1) one or more clinical events (eg, thrombocytopenia, thrombosis, disseminated intravascular coagulation [DIC], necrotizing skin lesions at heparin injection sites, post-intravenous heparin bolus anaphylactoid reaction) that bear a temporal association with a preceding immunizing heparin exposure; and (2) the presence of HIT-Abs (**Box 1**). Thus, a patient suspected to have HIT but in whom antibodies cannot be detected does not have this diagnosis. Rarely, patients develop a syndrome that mimics HIT on both clinical and serologic grounds but without a preceding exposure to heparin;[13–15] although named "spontaneous HIT," affected patients usually have a preceding inflammatory event such as infection or surgery.

Laboratory Testing for HIT-Abs

Detectability of HIT-Abs is a key diagnostic criterion. Properly performed, platelet activation assays (using washed platelets) and PF4-dependent enzyme immunoassays (EIAs) are very sensitive for HIT, and thus a negative assay generally rules out the diagnosis.[16] Platelet activation assays (eg, serotonin-release assay [SRA]) detect HIT-Abs based on their characteristic ability to activate platelets at therapeutic (0.1–0.3 U/mL) but not supratherapeutic (10–100 IU/mL) concentrations of UFH. More commonly, commercial PF4-dependent EIAs, which use PF4 bound to heparin or polyvinylsulfonate or platelet lysate proteins, are used to support a diagnosis of HIT.[16] However, approximately 15% to 25% of patients tested yield positive results in an immunoassay and, of these, only one-third to one-half also have a positive test for platelet-activating antibodies[16–18]; thus, only approximately 7% to 10% of patients who undergo serologic investigation for HIT truly have this diagnosis. In general, the more abnormal

---

Box 1

HIT: Clinical-pathologic criteria for diagnosis of HIT

Clinical

At least one of:

- Thrombocytopenia[a]

- Thrombosis (eg, *venous*: deep vein thrombosis, pulmonary embolism, venous limb gangrene, adrenal hemorrhage,[b] cerebral vein thrombosis, splanchnic vein thrombosis; *arterial*: limb artery thrombosis, stroke, myocardial infarction, mesenteric artery thrombosis, miscellaneous artery; *microvascular*)

- Necrotizing skin lesions at heparin injection sites[c]

- Acute anaphylactoid reactions[d]

Timing: above event(s) bear(s) temporal relation to a preceding immunizing heparin exposure[e]

Absence of another more compelling explanation

Pathologic

Heparin-dependent, platelet-activating IgG[f]

- Positive platelet activation assay (eg, serotonin-release assay)

- Positive anti-PF4/polyanion-IgG EIA (infers possibility of platelet-activating IgG)[g]

---

[a] >50% platelet count decrease is seen in ~90% of patients; in 5%–10%, the platelet decrease is 30%–50%.

[b] Adrenal hemorrhagic necrosis is a consequence of adrenal vein thrombosis.

[c] Nonnecrotizing lesions (erythematous plaques) are less specific for HIT.

[d] Usually occur 5–30 minutes after intravenous heparin bolus; rarely, after subcutaneous heparin.

[e] Typical-onset is 5–10 days after immunizing heparin exposure (usually given intra- or peri-operatively); rapid-onset HIT can occur if heparin is given to a patient who already has circulating HIT-Abs, usually due to heparin given in the last 5–100 days.

[f] Acute serum or plasma should be used for testing, as HIT-Abs are transient.

[g] In the appropriate context, a strong-positive EIA (IgG-specific or polyspecific assay that detects IgG/A/M antibodies) can be used to infer presence of platelet-activating HIT-Abs.

---

the test result (eg, higher percent serotonin release; higher optical density values in the EIA), the more likely it is the patient has HIT.[18] HIT-Abs are transient,[19] and thus acute serum or plasma should be tested.

FREQUENCY

The frequency of HIT varies widely, ranging from a negligible risk (eg, LMWH given during pregnancy) to a high of 5% to 10% (eg, females receiving UFH prophylaxis for 2 weeks after orthopedic surgery or during therapeutic-dose UFH post-implantation of a ventricular assist device).[20–23] PF4 and heparin form immunogenic complexes only at certain optimal ratios,[24] and thus stoichiometric considerations influence immunization risk (eg, postoperative patients with higher body mass index are more likely to form anti-PF4/heparin antibodies during fixed-dose prophylaxis with LMWH).[25] Other nondrug risk factors that appear to increase risk of HIT include trauma severity (the greater the degree of trauma, the more likely the patient is to develop anti-PF4/heparin antibodies and clinical HIT[26]) and the timing of heparin prophylaxis (eg, starting prophylaxis post- vs pre-surgery results in a higher frequency of antibody formation[25]).

PATHOGENESIS
Thrombin Generation

The central concept of HIT is formation of heparin-dependent antibodies of IgG isotype that activate platelets by causing signal transduction through platelet FcγIIa receptors.[27] The target antigen is a complex between (anionic) heparin and (cationic) PF4,[28,29] a tetrameric member of the CXC chemokine subfamily. HIT-Abs recognize conformationally altered sites on PF4 resulting from its binding to heparin[30] and/or because of close approximation of PF4 tetramers by heparin charge neutralization.[31] LMWH is less likely to trigger both antibodies and HIT, compared with UFH,[32,33] particularly in females receiving postsurgery thromboprophylaxis.[22] The pentasaccharide anticoagulant, fondaparinux, although similarly immunogenic as LMWH, does not form well the antigens on PF4,[34] suggesting it has an even lower risk of causing HIT.

HIT is a marked hypercoagulability state, as shown by greatly elevated markers of in vivo thrombin generation, for example, thrombin-antithrombin complexes.[6] The explanation for extreme hypercoagulability is uncertain, but could represent pancellular activation,[35] including formation of prothrombotic platelet-derived microparticles,[36] as well as tissue factor expression through activation of monocytes.[37]

The "Timeline" of HIT

The temporal features of antibody formation are consistent with a "point" immunization when heparin is given under circumstances that favor immunization.[38–40] One such setting is surgery (release of PF4 of activated platelets; perioperative inflammation). HIT-Ab levels first become detectable 4 days (median) after intra- or postoperative heparin administration, followed by the beginning of the HIT-associated platelet count decrease 2 days later (median, day 6) followed by reaching a large-magnitude (>50%) platelet count decrease 2 days later (median, day 8).[40] On average, thrombotic events occur 2 to 3 days later (median, day 10–11), but sometimes occur shortly before the beginning of the platelet count decrease.[2] Antibody levels typically peak between days 10 and 14,[39,40] and in some patients the platelet count can continue to decrease—or even *begin* to decrease—after cessation of heparin ("delayed-onset" HIT).[41–43] Of note, after reaching their peak HIT-Ab levels can decline even with continued heparin administration.[39]

THERAPY

The 6 treatment principles of HIT can be summarized as: "2 *Do's*," "2 *Don'ts*," and "2 *Diagnostics*" (**Box 2**).[44] A crucial tenet is avoiding/postponing warfarin.[3,4,6]

Warfarin is Contraindicated During Acute HIT

Acute HIT is a major risk factor for warfarin (coumarin) necrosis, which can manifest either as venous limb gangrene or classic skin necrosis.[6,38,45–48] The pathogenesis is microthrombosis due to depletion of protein C (vitamin K-dependent natural anticoagulant) in the setting of increased thrombin generation from HIT, that is, disturbed procoagulant-anticoagulant balance.[6,48]

Venous limb gangrene is characterized by: (1) an underlying hypercoagulability state such as HIT; (2) acral (distal extremity) necrosis in a limb affected by deep vein thrombosis (DVT); and (3) a supratherapeutic international normalized ratio (INR) usually >3.5 (representing a surrogate marker for severe protein C depletion).[6,48,49] In contrast, classic warfarin-induced skin necrosis features involvement of skin and subcutaneous tissues at central (nonacral) sites, for example, breast, abdomen, thigh, calf.[48,50]

Box 2
Six treatment principles for management of confirmed or strongly suspected HIT

Principle	Comment
Two Do's	
Do stop all heparin, including heparin "flushes" and LMWH[a]	Paradoxically, stopping heparin can *worsen* risk of thrombosis, because heparin is anticoagulant and HIT-Abs can activate platelets even in its absence
Do give an alternative nonheparin anticoagulant (therapeutic-dose)[b]	Heparin cessation alone is frequently complicated by thrombotic complications
Two Don'ts	
Don't give warfarin (give vitamin K if warfarin has already been given)	Warfarin does not block HIT hypercoagulability, increases microthrombosis risk via protein C depletion, and leads to underdosing of APTT-adjusted DTI therapy
Don't give platelet transfusions	Thrombocytopenic bleeding is uncommon in HIT, and platelets might increase risk for thrombosis
Two Diagnostics	
Test for HIT-Abs	Negative tests rule out HIT; strong-positive tests[c] are usually seen in "true" HIT
Image for lower-limb DVT	DVT is the most common complication of HIT

Abbreviations: DTI, direct thrombin inhibitor; DVT, deep vein thrombosis; HIT-Abs, HIT antibodies; LMWH, low-molecular-weight heparin; APTT, activated partial thromboplastin time.
[a] Continuation of heparin (including LMWH) as a therapeutic option is unexplored.
[b] Danaparoid, fondaparinux, lepirudin, argatroban, bivalirudin (usually in therapeutic doses).
[c] Anti-PF4/polyanion enzyme immunoassay; serotonin-release assay.

The risk of coumarin necrosis in HIT is approximately 5% to 10%,[6] a frequency much greater than the background risk (overall, ~0.01%).[50] Vitamin K is recommended if a diagnosis of HIT is made after warfarin has already been started,[3,4,47,51] which is aimed to avoid systematic underdosing of DTIs when their therapy is monitored using the activated partial thromboplastin time (APTT),[47] as the APTT is prolonged by warfarin.

A Conceptual Approach to Therapy for HIT

Fig. 1 illustrates key concepts in the management of HIT. The top panel shows the typical "timeline" of HIT-Ab seroconversion.[39,40] HIT-Ab levels continue to increase after stopping heparin, and typically peak 10 to 14 days after the immunizing heparin exposure. Thus, platelet count declines—and associated hypercoagulability—can intensify despite stopping heparin, and worsen thrombotic events, often manifesting as progressive microvascular thrombosis that complicates preceding macrovascular thrombosis. For example, a patient with HIT-associated DVT can develop venous limb gangrene as a result of progressive microvascular thrombosis, or a patient with HIT-associated arterial thrombosis can develop ischemic limb necrosis—even after embolectomy—because of progressive microvascular thrombosis in the affected limb.

There are several reasons why thrombosis risk is very high during the days 7 to 14 time period: (1) loss of heparin's anticoagulant effect (including, paradoxically, the iatrogenic factor of stopping heparin because of thrombocytopenia recognition); (2) progressive increase in HIT-Ab levels,[39,40] often with substantial

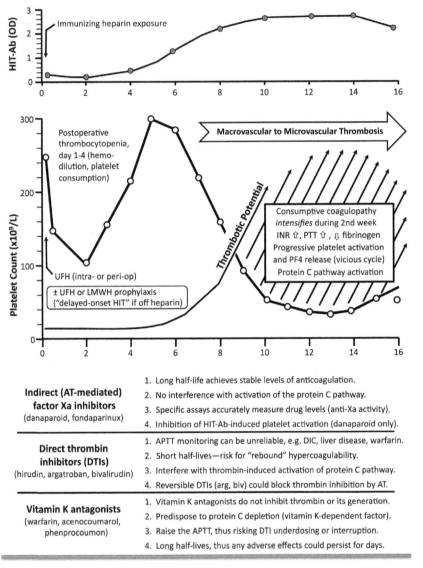

Indirect (AT-mediated) factor Xa inhibitors (danaparoid, fondaparinux)	1. Long half-life achieves stable levels of anticoagulation.
	2. No interference with activation of the protein C pathway.
	3. Specific assays accurately measure drug levels (anti-Xa activity).
	4. Inhibition of HIT-Ab-induced platelet activation (danaparoid only).
Direct thrombin inhibitors (DTIs) (hirudin, argatroban, bivalirudin)	1. APTT monitoring can be unreliable, e.g. DIC, liver disease, warfarin.
	2. Short half-lives—risk for "rebound" hypercoagulability.
	3. Interfere with thrombin-induced activation of protein C pathway.
	4. Reversible DTIs (arg, biv) could block thrombin inhibition by AT.
Vitamin K antagonists (warfarin, acenocoumarol, phenprocoumon)	1. Vitamin K antagonists do not inhibit thrombin or its generation.
	2. Predispose to protein C depletion (vitamin K-dependent factor).
	3. Raise the APTT, thus risking DTI underdosing or interruption.
	4. Long half-lives, thus any adverse effects could persist for days.

Fig. 1. Conceptual framework of HIT. The upper panel shows the timeline of HIT antibody (HIT-Ab) formation, as judged by optical density units in an anti-PF4/polyanion EIA; the middle panel illustrates the typical platelet count profile, and indicates that intensification of HIT-associated hypercoagulability occurs from day 7 to 14, especially after stopping heparin. The lower panel compares different classes of anticoagulant for expected effects on HIT-associated hypercoagulability.

heparin-independent platelet-activating properties,[41,52,53] that is, platelet activation can intensify for several days after stopping heparin; (3) progressive release of PF4 from activated platelets, leading to greater formation of PF4/polyanion complexes on platelet surfaces (self-enhancing vicious cycle),[54] producing greater platelet activation, procoagulant microparticle formation, and increased thrombin generation.

DTIs have potential drawbacks that could limit their effectiveness during this period of intense HIT-associated hypercoagulability. Global coagulation assays (eg, APTT) used to monitor their effects may give misleading information.[47] Also, due to their short half-lives, dose reduction or drug cessation can lead to "rebound" hypercoagulability.[55]

Another issue is potential interference by DTIs of activation of the protein C anticoagulant pathway, which is needed to down-regulate thrombin in HIT-associated hypercoagulability. Warfarin anticoagulation—with protein C depletion—is an important factor explaining microvascular complications in approximately 90% of patients who develop venous limb gangrene in HIT.[6,45] In theory, DTIs could also promote microvascular thrombosis in certain circumstances, either through inhibiting thrombin-mediated activation of protein C, or (for reversible DTIs, argatroban and bivalirudin) by impeding AT3-mediated inhibition of thrombin. Indeed, cases of venous limb gangrene during DTI-warfarin overlap suggest this period is fraught with risk of progressive microvascular thrombosis.[46,47]

The bottom panel of **Fig. 1** compares the indirect (AT3-mediated) inhibitors of factor Xa with DTIs and vitamin K antagonists. Various factors supporting the advantages of the Xa inhibitors vis-à-vis the other 2 drug classes are summarized.

NONHEPARIN ANTICOAGULANTS
Anticoagulants for HIT: the Main Five Agents

Three nonheparin anticoagulants, danaparoid, lepirudin, and argatroban, are approved for treatment of HIT, although approvals vary by jurisdiction. Two other agents, fondaparinux and bivalirudin, are marketed for non-HIT indications, but have a biologic rationale for HIT therapy. These 5 drugs can be classified into 2 groups: those with long-acting AT3-dependent inhibition of factor Xa (danaparoid, fondaparinux) and the AT3-independent DTIs (r-hirudin, argatroban, bivalirudin). **Box 3** summarizes key differences between these 2 groups, emphasizing specific implications for HIT. As indicated by the "check marks" ($\sqrt{}$), the Xa-inhibiting drugs have several advantages over DTIs for management of HIT.

Long-acting AT3-dependent Inhibitors of Factor Xa: Danaparoid and Fondaparinux

Danaparoid
Danaparoid is a mixture of anticoagulant glycosaminoglycans, predominantly low-sulfated heparan sulfate.[7] Danaparoid has both anti-thrombin and anti-Xa activity, although the latter predominates (anti-Xa/anti-thrombin ratio, ~22). The half-life of its anti-Xa activity is approximately 25 hours. Danaparoid can be given by both subcutaneous and intravenous injection, although the American College of Chest Physicians (ACCP) Evidence-Based Clinical Practice Guidelines (8th edition) recommends that it be given at least initially by intravenous bolus to ensure rapid attainment of therapeutic concentrations.[3,4] An intriguing property of danaparoid is that, at therapeutic concentrations, it *inhibits* HIT-Ab-induced platelet activation in a large percentage of HIT sera.[56] Theoretically, agents such as 2-O, 3-O desulfated heparin[57] could also be used to inhibit platelet activation.

Danaparoid is approved both for HIT and/or non-HIT indications in several jurisdictions, including Canada, Europe, Australia, New Zealand, and Japan; notably, it is not approved for management of HIT in the United States, and has not been available in that market since 2002. Beginning in early 2009, manufacturing problems led to shortages, and the drug continues to have limited availability in some markets.

Danaparoid for treatment of HIT Danaparoid is the only agent evaluated in a randomized controlled trial for management of HIT. Here, it was superior to the comparator

Box 3
A comparison of 2 classes of anticoagulant used to treat HIT

	Indirect AT3-Dependent Factor Xa Inhibitors: Danaparoid, Fondaparinux	Direct AT3-Independent Thrombin Inhibitors: r-Hirudin, Argatroban, Bivalirudin
Half-life	√ Long (>16 h): avoids potential for rebound hypercoagulability	Short (<2 h): potential for rebound hypercoagulability
Dosing	√ Both prophylactic- and therapeutic-dose regimens[a]	Prophylactic-dose regimens are not established
Monitoring	√ Direct (anti-Xa levels): accurate drug levels obtained	Indirect (APTT): risk for DTI underdosing due to APTT elevation for non-DTI factors
Effect on INR	√ No significant effect: thus, simplifies overlap with warfarin	Increases INR: argatroban > bivalirudin > r-hirudin; complicates warfarin overlap
Protein C pathway	√ No significant effect	Thrombin inhibition could impair activation of protein C pathway
Reversibility of action	√ Irreversible inhibition (AT3 forms covalent bond to Xa)	Irreversible inhibition only with r-hirudin
Platelet activation	√ Danaparoid inhibits platelet activation by HIT-Abs	No effect
Drug clearance	Predominantly renal	Variable (see text)

Check mark indicates positive feature in comparison of drug classes.
[a] Although therapeutic dosing recommended for HIT, availability of prophylactic-dose regimens increases flexibility when managing potential non-HIT situations.

agent, dextran-70.[58] This trial consisted of danaparoid plus warfarin versus dextran-70 plus warfarin. If one assumes that dextran has minimal anticoagulant activity, the comparator essentially consisted of warfarin alone. This design resembles somewhat that of a retrospective study of danaparoid versus comparators that included ancrod and/or coumarin.[59] Pooling these 2 studies (**Table 1**), danaparoid appears efficacious for HIT. Indeed, danaparoid is the *only* anticoagulant evaluated for HIT that in comparison with a control group, showed a significantly lower thrombotic rate while at the same time showing a significantly lower major bleeding rate. A retrospective comparison[60] of lepirudin with danaparoid suggested that prophylactic-dose danaparoid is less effective than lepirudin, whereas therapeutic-dose danaparoid showed efficacy broadly comparable to that of lepirudin (see **Table 1**).

In the author's opinion, useful information can be obtained from careful observational studies of treatment outcomes in patients with severe HIT. For example, ancrod (defibrinogenating snake venom) was first thought to be effective for HIT treatment.[61] However, on greater use—including in patients with severe HIT—it became apparent that this therapy often failed.[59] In contrast, the author has used danaparoid in many patients with severe HIT, with excellent results. **Fig. 2** shows a dramatic example: this patient had overt DIC and bilateral foot microvascular ischemia at the time of referral, and developed the lowest platelet count ever observed by the author in HIT (2×10^9/L). Therapeutic-dose danaparoid was administered, which was stopped one weekend by a physician who decided to stop anticoagulation because of the severe thrombocytopenia! Fortunately, the long half-life helped maintain drug levels

Table 1
Selected studies of danaparoid for treatment of HIT

Study	New Thrombosis	Limb Amputation	Composite End Point[a]	Major Bleeds
Chong et al, 2001[58]	Dan: 3/24 (12.5%)	Dan: 1/24 (4.2%)	Dan: 6/24 (25.0%)	Dan: 0/24 (0%)
	Ctrl: 7/17 (41.2%)	Ctrl: 3/17 (17.6%)	Ctrl: 10/17 (58.8%)	Ctrl: 0/17 (0%)
	RR = 0.30 (0.09, 1.01)	RR = 0.24 (0.03, 2.08)	RR = 0.43 (0.19, 0.94)	$P = 1.0$
	$P = .063$	$P = .29$	$P = .050$	
Lubenow et al, 2006[59]	Dan: 11/62 (17.7%)	Dan: 3/62 (4.8%)	Dan: 15/62 (24.2%)	Dan: 8/62 (12.9%)
	Ctrl: 24/56 (42.9%)	Ctrl: 4/56 (7.1%)	Ctrl: 28/56 (50.0%)	Ctrl: 19/56 (33.9%)
	RR = 0.41 (0.22, 0.77)[b]	RR = 0.68 (0.16, 2.90)	RR = 0.48 (0.29, 0.81)	RR = 0.38 (0.18, 0.80)[b]
	$P = .0044$	$P = .71$	$P = .0043$	$P = .0084$
Refs.[58,59] (pooled[c])	Dan: 14/86 (16.3%)	Dan: 4/86 (4.7%)	Dan: 21/86 (24.4%)	Dan: 8/86 (9.3%)
	Ctrl: 31/73 (42.5%)	Ctrl: 7/73 (9.6%)	Ctrl: 38/73 (52.1%)	Ctrl: 19/73 (26.0%)
	RR = 0.38 (0.22, 0.66)[b]	RR = 0.48 (0.15, 1.59)	RR = 0.47 (0.30, 0.72)	RR = 0.36 (0.17, 0.77)[b]
	$P = .00036$	$P = .35$	$P = .0005$	$P = .0060$
Farner et al, 2001[60,d]	Dan: 5/53 (9.4%)	Dan: 4/53 (7.5%)	Dan: 10/53 (18.9%)	Dan: 2/53 (3.8%)
	Lep: 9/114 (7.9%)	Lep: 7/114 (6.1%)	Lep: 21/114 (18.4%)	Lep: 7/114 (6.1%)
	RR = 1.20 (0.42, 3.39)	RR = 1.23 (0.38, 4.02)	RR = 1.02 (0.52, 2.02)	RR = 0.62 (0.13, 2.86)
	$P = .77$	$P = .74$	$P = 1.0$	$P = .72$

Abbreviations: Ctrl, control; Dan, danaparoid.

[a] Composite end point: all-cause mortality, all-cause limb amputation, and/or new thrombosis (each patient counted only once).

[b] Danaparoid is the only anticoagulant evaluated for HIT that showed significantly greater efficacy and reduced bleeding, compared with a control group.

[c] The rationale for pooling includes similar nature of control groups.

[d] Only patients who received therapeutic-dose danaparoid patients are included.

Data from Tables 5a and 5b in Warkentin TE, Greinacher A, Koster A, et al. Treatment and prevention of heparin-induced thrombocytopenia. American College of Chest Physicians evidence-based clinical practice guidelines (8th edition). Chest 2008;133(Suppl 6):340S–80S.

for several hours despite its cessation, and the danaparoid was resumed on Monday morning without adverse events. This case also illustrates that accurate drug levels (anti-Xa levels) can be achieved in the setting of overt DIC, which is not possible using the APTT—the most common test for monitoring DTI therapy.

Fondaparinux

Fondaparinux is an indirect (AT3-dependent) inhibitor of factor Xa modeled after the pentasaccharide region of heparin.[11] Fondaparinux shares several similarities with danaparoid. Both have anti–factor Xa activity, either exclusively (fondaparinux) or predominantly (danaparoid). Both fondaparinux and danaparoid have long anti–factor Xa half-lives (17 and 25 hours, respectively), and both show either absent (fondaparinux) or absent/weak (danaparoid) in vitro cross-reactivity with HIT antibodies.[34] As

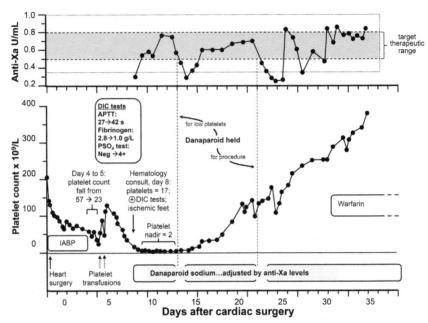

Fig. 2. Danaparoid for very severe HIT. Despite overt DIC, bilateral limb ischemia, and the lowest platelet count (2×10^9/L) due to HIT encountered by the author, this patient fully recovered from HIT and without loss of limbs or any other permanent sequelae. The evidence for overt DIC included: elevated APTT, reduced fibrinogen, and strongly positive (4+) protamine sulfate (PSO_4) paracoagulation assay at day 8, which represents changes from normal values at day 5. IABP, intra-aortic balloon pump.

fondaparinux is marketed in a prophylactic-dose regimen (2.5 mg once daily) for prevention of thrombosis after orthopedic surgery, this suggests that it also may be appropriate for prevention of thrombosis in its low-dose regimen in non-HIT situations in which the physician would prefer not to give heparin, for example, a thrombocytopenic patient in whom HIT is judged unlikely.[4] As with danaparoid, therapeutic dosing is likely required to treat severe HIT.

Does putative fondaparinux-associated HIT have implications for its use in treatment of HIT? An intriguing issue is that 3 cases of HIT have been reported during fondaparinux thromboprophylaxis post orthopedic surgery.[62–64] Serologic studies of one case showed the HIT-Abs activated platelets in the absence of heparin, and without increase in platelet activation with fondaparinux. These findings are consistent with observations[34] showing *dissociation* between immunogenicity and cross-reactivity of anti-PF4/heparin antibodies: whereas fondaparinux is associated with formation of anti-PF4/heparin antibodies (at a frequency similar to that of the LMWH, enoxaparin), it usually does not promote binding of the antibodies to PF4 (ie, unlike LMWH, fondaparinux does not exhibit cross-reactivity). The implications are that fondaparinux—at therapeutic concentrations—should be an effective therapy even for patients who develop HIT during fondaparinux prophylaxis! The author's view is that the rare reports of fondaparinux as a cause of the HIT syndrome do not argue against it being, potentially, an effective agent to manage HIT, irrespective of its trigger.

Fondaparinux for the treatment of HIT **Table 2** lists 3 observational studies[65–67] evaluating fondaparinux for management of acute HIT (minimum, 5 patients per study). None of the studies used a platelet activation assay to confirm the diagnosis of HIT.

Table 2
Fondaparinux for treatment of acute HIT: studies of 5 or more patients

Study	N	HIT-T	Median Platelet Count Nadir, ×10⁹/L (Range)	EIA Results[a] (OD Units)	Dose[b]	Thrombosis Rate	Amputation Rate	Major Bleeding Rate
Kuo and Kovacs, 2005[65]	5	5/5	56 (5, 79)	>1.0 in all 5	7.5 mg	0/5	0/5	0/5
Lobo et al, 2008[66]	7	6/7[c]	67 (11, 139)	0.7 (median)	7.5 mg[d]	0/7	1/7[e]	0/7
Grouzi et al, 2010[67]	24	14/24[f]	66[g] (N.A.)	1.4 (mean)[h]	7.5 mg	0/24	1/24[i]	0/24
Pooled	36	25/36 (69.4%)	~65[j]	>1.0 (median)	7.5 mg	0/36 (0%)	2/36 (5.6%)	0/36 (0%)

A PubMed search performed on January 10, 2010 using "fondaparinux" and "heparin-induced thrombocytopenia" had 116 "hits," "from which 3 articles were identified that described the use of fondaparinux for 5 or more cases of acute HIT.

Abbreviations: EIA, enzyme immunoassay; HIT-T, HIT-associated thrombosis (ie, patients who developed thrombosis in association with developing HIT); N.A., not available; OD, optical density.

[a] All patients tested EIA-positive; no patients were tested in a platelet activation assay.
[b] Dose per day administered by subcutaneous injection (10 mg and 5 mg if the patient weighed >100 kg and <50 kg, respectively).
[c] One patient had thrombosis that preceded HIT; the other 6 patients had HIT-associated thrombosis (HIT-T).
[d] The single patient without HIT-T received 2.5 mg daily by subcutaneous injection.
[e] One patient with popliteal artery thrombosis and failed thrombectomy required amputation; however, the ischemic limb necrosis was judged to have been present before fondaparinux therapy.
[f] All 10 patients without HIT-T nevertheless had preceding thrombosis that led to the heparin therapy that triggered HIT.
[g] The platelet count nadir excludes 2 patients with myeloproliferative disease and baseline thrombocytosis.
[h] The mean OD was significantly greater (2.0 units) in the 14 patients with HIT-T.
[i] One patient had limb amputation before commencing fondaparinux.
[j] Estimated median platelet count nadir of the 34 patients (excluding 2 with myeloproliferative disease).

However, it appears the majority of patients really had HIT, based on: (1) the median platelet count ($\sim$65); (2) all 36 patients had a positive EIA, usually a strong positive result (>1.0 optical density units); (3) 69% had putative HIT-associated thrombosis.

The pooled results are impressive: no patient developed new thrombosis (0/36; upper 95% limit, 8.0%), and none had major bleeding. Although 2 patients underwent limb amputations, these appeared because of limb necrosis that preceded fondaparinux use; further, the overall frequency of limb amputation ($\sim$5.0%) was similar to that of 2 other effective treatments for HIT (danaparoid, lepirudin), suggesting that 5% may be a practical "lower limit" for limb amputation in HIT that reflects rapid and irreversible ischemic limb injury for which no effective therapy is possible.

Direct Thrombin Inhibitors

Table 3 compares and contrasts DTIs that have been used for the treatment of HIT.

r-Hirudin

Two r-hirudins, lepirudin (Refludan) and desirudin (Iprivask in the United States, Revasc elsewhere), are marketed, although only lepirudin is approved for anticoagulation of patients with HIT and associated thromboembolic disease. Despite its noncovalent nature, the very high affinity of r-hirudin for thrombin results in essentially irreversible binding. Lepirudin reduces thrombin generation in HIT.[8] Its elimination is through renal clearance.

Dosing of lepirudin An important issue is that the Food and Drug Administration (FDA)-approved dosing (per package insert) is substantially higher than that recommended by consensus conference guidelines[4] based on 4 studies[68–71] concluding that the approved therapeutic-dose regimen leads to a high frequency (15%–20%) of major bleeding, including fatal bleeding rates of 2.4% to 3.9%,[69,71] without reduced efficacy among those achieving therapeutic versus supratherapeutic drug levels. Risk increases further even with mild renal dysfunction.

Therapeutic efficacy of lepirudin Table 4 shows pooled data from the approval studies of lepirudin[69] and argatroban[72–74] for treatment of HIT-associated thrombosis. Compared with historical controls, lepirudin appears highly efficacious. The relative risk (RR) of thrombosis was 0.28, that is, the rate of new thrombosis in lepirudin-treated patients was 7%, compared with 25% control rate. This came at a cost, however: the frequency of major bleeding with lepirudin was 15%, compared with 7% in controls (RR, 2.31; $P = .072$).

Argatroban

Argatroban is FDA-approved for the prevention or treatment of thrombosis associated with HIT. Argatroban's affinity for thrombin is greater than 4-log lower than that of lepirudin (K_i, 40 vs 0.0001 nmol/L) and, unlike hirudin, its binding to thrombin is reversible. Argatroban is primarily eliminated through hepatobiliary clearance.

Therapeutic efficacy of argatroban Table 4 summarizes pooled data from the approval studies of argatroban for the treatment of HIT-associated thrombosis. Compared with historical controls, argatroban had an RR of 0.45, that is, the rate of new thrombosis in argatroban-treated patients was 16%, compared with 35% frequency in controls. The frequency of major bleeding in argatroban-treated patients was 8%, compared with only 2% in controls, an RR of 3.70 ($P = .231$).

Argatroban and limb amputations The pooled data summarized in **Table 4** show that there is a relatively high limb amputation rate (14%) in patients with HIT-associated

Table 3
Comparison of DTIs used for treatment of HIT

	r-Hirudin	Argatroban	Bivalirudin
Structure	Lepirudin (65-a.a., 6980 Da) and desirudin (65-a.a. 6960 Da) are recombinant derivatives of hirudin (leech anticoagulant)[a]	Small-molecule arginine derivative (527 Da)	C-terminal hirudin region linked by polyglycine spacer to tetrapeptide reactive with thrombin active site (20-a.a., 2180 Da)
Anticoagulant action	High affinity (K_i = 0.0001 nmol/L) and *irreversible* binding to 2 sites on thrombin, ie, *bivalent* DTI	Moderate affinity (K_i = 40 nmol/L) and *reversible* binding to active site of thrombin (*univalent* DTI)	Moderate to high affinity (K_i = 1.9–2.3 nmol/L) and reversible[b] binding to active site of thrombin (*bivalent* DTI)
Immunologic features	No effect on HIT Ab-induced platelet activation; lepirudin is immunogenic (allergic/anaphylactic reactions are reported)	No effect on HIT Ab-induced platelet activation; nonimmunogenic (cf lepirudin)	No effect on HIT Ab-induced platelet activation; potentially cross-reactive with antihirudin antibodies
Half-life	80 min (normal renal function)	40–50 min (normal hepatobiliary function)	25 min (enzymic metabolism)
Dosing regimen	No bolus; initial rate, 0.10 mg/kg/h[c] (adjust to APTT[d]); reduce dose for renal dysfunction[e]	No bolus; initial rate, 0.5–2 μg/kg/min[f] (adjust to APTT[d]); reduce in liver disease[g]	Not established; no bolus; initial dose, 0.15–0.20 mg/kg/h has been suggested[4]
Clearance	Renal	Hepatobiliary[g]	Enzymic; renal (minor)
Monitoring	APTT[d]	APTT[d]	APTT[d]

Abbreviations: a.a., amino acid; Ab, antibody; APTT, activated partial thromboplastin time; Da, Daltons; DIC, disseminated intravascular coagulation.

[a] Compared with natural hirudin, both lepirudin and desirudin are desulfated at Tyr_{63}, which results in tenfold reduced affinity for thrombin compared with natural hirudin (not clinically significant); the molecular mass difference between lepirudin and desirudin is explained by one difference in a.a. composition: Leu_1 (lepirudin) compared with Ile_1 (desirudin).

[b] The initial binding between bivalirudin and thrombin is specific and noncompetitive. However, thrombin can cleave the Arg_3-Pro_4 of bivalirudin, following which bivalirudin's N-terminal sequence no longer binds to thrombin, leaving the residual C-terminal dodecapeptide with greatly reduced binding affinity for exosite 1 of thrombin, thus transforming bivalirudin into a competitive, and reversible, inhibitor of thrombin.

[c] This dosing regimen is much lower than that described in the manufacturer's package insert.

[d] The APTT is not reliable for anticoagulant monitoring in patients with preexisting congenital or acquired coagulopathies, overt DIC, prolonged APTT due to "lupus anticoagulant," or effects of warfarin; methods for measuring drug levels directly are available in some jurisdictions (especially in Europe).

[e] The initial lepirudin infusion rate should be no higher than 0.10 mg/kg/h (serum creatinine <90 μmol/L), with lower infusion rates for patients with higher serum creatinine levels (90–140 μmol/L, start at 0.05 mg/kg/h; 140–400, start at 0.01 mg/kg/h; >400, start at 0.005 mg/kg/h). APTT monitoring should be performed at 4-h intervals until it is apparent that steady state within the therapeutic range (1.5–2.5 times patient baseline [or mean laboratory] APTT) has been achieved.

[f] Although manufacturer's package insert recommends that dosing start at 2 μg/kg/min, many clinicians start at lower doses, eg, 0.5–1.2 μg/kg/min, especially in patients who are critically ill or who have cardiac failure.

[g] For patients with moderate or greater liver dysfunction, the starting dose is 0.5 μg/kg/min.

Table 4
Summary of studies describing efficacy of the DTIs (lepirudin, argatroban) as treatment for thrombosis complicating HIT

Study	Intervention	New Thrombosis	Amputation Rate	Composite End Point[a]	Major Bleeds	Comment
Lubenow et al, 2005[69]	Lep: bolus, 0.4 mg/kg; 0.15 mg/kg/h[b] Con: variable	Lep: 15/214 (7%) Con: 19/75 (25%) RR = 0.28 (0.15, 0.52) P<.001	Lep: 12/214 (6%) Con: 6/75 (8%) RR = 0.70 (0.27, 1.80) P = .58	Lep: 41/214 (19%) Con: 30/75 (40%) RR = 0.48 (0.32, 0.71) P<.001	Lep: 33/214 (15%)[c] Con: 5/75 (7%) RR = 2.31 (0.94, 5.71) P = .072	All patients tested positive for HIT-Abs; data are pooled from 3 studies versus historical controls
Lewis et al, 2001, 2003, 2006[72–74]	Arg: 2 µg/kg/min (no bolus)[d] Con: variable (eg, coumarin)	Arg: 58/373 (16%) Con: 16/46 (35%) RR = 0.45 (0.28, 0.71) P = .0032	Arg: 51/373 (14%) Con: 5/46 (11%) RR = 1.26 (0.53, 2.99) P = .81	Arg: 158/373 (42%) Con: 26/46 (57%) RR = 0.75 (0.57, 0.99) P = .083	Arg: 30/373 (8%)[c] Con: 1/46 (2%) RR = 3.70 (0.52, 26.50) P = .231	Patients did not require positive test for HIT-Abs[e]; data are pooled from 3 studies versus historical controls

95% confidence intervals are provided for RRs (risk ratios); P values are Fisher's exact test, 2-tailed, unless otherwise indicated.

Abbreviations: APTT, activated partial thromboplastin time; Arg, argatroban; Con, control; HIPA, heparin-induced platelet activation; Lep, lepirudin.

[a] Composite end point: all-cause mortality, all-cause limb amputation, and/or new thrombosis (each patient counted only once).

[b] APTT adjusted to 1.5–2.5 times baseline APTT (or mean of laboratory APTT range); mean treatment duration was 15.8 days (for 214 lepirudin-treated patients).

[c] Major bleeding, expressed *per treatment day*, was 0.97% for lepirudin and 1.25% for argatroban.

[d] APTT adjusted to 1.5–3.0 times baseline APTT; mean argatroban treatment duration was 6.6 days (for 373 argatroban-treated patients).

[e] 65% of argatroban-treated patients tested positive for HIT antibodies in Arg-911 study[71] (data not available for the Arg-915/915X studies[72]).

Data from Table 4a in Warkentin TE, Greinacher A, Koster A, et al. Treatment and prevention of heparin-induced thrombocytopenia. American College of Chest Physicians evidence-based clinical practice guidelines (8th edition). Chest 2008;133(Suppl 6):340S–80S.

thrombosis treated with argatroban. This frequency seems higher than the approximately 5% "floor" rate observed with lepirudin, danaparoid, and fondaparinux. Possible factors to explain the high limb loss rate with argatroban could include: (1) difficulty in identifying an appropriate therapeutic drug level; (2) problems of argatroban-warfarin overlap (argatroban raises the INR more than does bivalirudin and lepirudin, potentially complicating warfarin overlap)[75]; (3) its reversible binding to thrombin (theoretical potential for impaired AT-mediated thrombin neutralization); (4) the high molar concentrations required to prolong the APTT[75] could impair protein C pathway activation; and (5) its relatively short half-life could lead to a higher frequency of rebound hypercoagulability if the drug is stopped prematurely.

Fig. 3 illustrates difficulties in achieving a therapeutic concentration. Here, numerous argatroban dose interruptions/resumptions occurred while aiming to achieve a therapeutic drug level. Also, the baseline elevated APTT raises the issue of whether the later "therapeutic" APTT levels truly reflected adequate drug levels, or whether instead the APTT prolongation indicated subtherapeutic levels in a patient with other reasons for APTT increase.

Bivalirudin

Bivalirudin is 1 of the 5 anticoagulants listed by the ACCP consensus conference as a rational therapy for HIT,[4,51] though experience is limited. Further, many of the

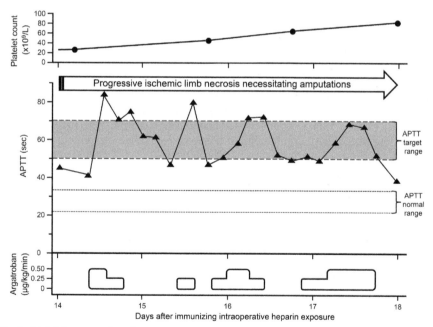

Fig. 3. Multiple argatroban dose interruptions and resumptions during DTI therapy. Two "baseline" (pre-argatroban) APTT values were elevated (45.1 and 41.4 seconds). The normal APTT range was 22 to 34 seconds, which was used to determine the "therapeutic range" of 50 to 70 seconds (approximately 2–3 times the midpoint of the normal laboratory APTT range); however, this could have an inappropriately low target range, given the patient's elevated baseline APTT representing either HIT-associated consumptive coagulopathy or hepatic dysfunction. Because the pre-argatroban transaminases were approximately tenfold elevated, the patient was deemed to have liver disease, and so the initial dose of argatroban was 0.5 μg/kg/min. The multiple dose interruptions and resumptions could have contributed to the adverse outcome.

patients treated with bivalirudin have had renal or hepatic failure (or even both), limiting conclusions given that this population has a high mortality rate. Indeed, as bivalirudin exhibits substantial nonrenal/nonhepatic clearance—through enzymic degradation—there is some rationale for its use in critically ill patients.[76]

Direct measurement of plasma DTI levels

Commercial methods have become available to assay DTI drug levels directly, although these are not currently in wide use. Accurate drug levels could improve clinical outcomes, particularly in situations whereby indirect monitoring (APTT) yields misleading results.

REPEAT HEPARIN EXPOSURE FOR PATIENTS WITH PREVIOUS HIT

For patients with a previous history of HIT who have an important indication for heparin (eg, cardiac or vascular surgery), it is recommended to use heparin, provided that HIT-Abs are no longer detectable, or (in emergencies) that sufficient time has passed so that clinically significant levels of HIT-Abs are not likely to be present. This advice is given because a previous history of HIT does not appear to be a risk factor for a higher frequency of forming HIT-Abs during subsequent exposure, and in any event such antibodies would not regenerate in high levels for at least 5 days, at which time a non-heparin anticoagulant can be used.

SUMMARY

Long-activating inhibitors of factor Xa, danaparoid and fondaparinux, have several advantages over DTIs for management of HIT, including their long half-life, their lack of interference with protein C pathway, and the availability of specific assays to permit accurate determination of drug levels. Particularly during the intense period of HIT-associated hypercoagulability, which is seen approximately 7 to 14 days after the immunizing heparin exposure, effective anticoagulation is needed to prevent micro-vascular thrombosis from contributing to tissue ischemic necrosis that often occurs in the setting of preceding macrovascular thrombosis.

ACKNOWLEDGMENTS

Thanks to Jo-Ann I. Sheppard for preparation of the figures.

REFERENCES

1. Warkentin TE, Kelton JG. A 14-year study of heparin-induced thrombocytopenia. Am J Med 1996;101(5):502–7.
2. Greinacher A, Farner B, Kroll H, et al. Clinical features of heparin-induced thrombocytopenia including risk factors for thrombosis. A retrospective analysis of 408 patients. Thromb Haemost 2005;94(1):132–5.
3. Warkentin TE, Greinacher A. Heparin-induced thrombocytopenia: recognition, treatment, and prevention. The seventh ACCP conference on antithrombotic and thrombolytic therapy. Chest 2004;126(Suppl 3):311S–37S.
4. Warkentin TE, Greinacher A, Koster A, et al. Treatment and prevention of heparin-induced thrombocytopenia. American College of Chest Physicians evidence-based clinical practice guidelines (8th edition). Chest 2008;133(Suppl 6): 340S–80S.

5. Wallis DE, Workman DL, Lewis BE, et al. Failure of early heparin cessation as treatment for heparin-induced thrombocytopenia. Am J Med 1999;106(6): 629–35.

6. Warkentin TE, Elavathil LJ, Hayward CPM, et al. The pathogenesis of venous limb gangrene associated with heparin-induced thrombocytopenia. Ann Intern Med 1997;127(9):804–12.

7. Chong BH, Magnani HN. Danaparoid for the treatment of heparin-induced thrombocytopenia. In: Warkentin TE, Greinacher A, editors. Heparin-induced thrombocytopenia. 4th edition. New York: Informa Healthcare USA, Inc; 2007. p. 319–43.

8. Greinacher A. Lepirudin for the treatment of heparin-induced thrombocytopenia. In: Warkentin TE, Greinacher A, editors. Heparin-induced thrombocytopenia. 4th edition. New York: Informa Healthcare USA, Inc; 2007. p. 345–78.

9. Lewis BE, Hursting MJ. Argatroban therapy in heparin-induced thrombocytopenia. In: Warkentin TE, Greinacher A, editors. Heparin-induced thrombocytopenia. 4th edition. New York: Informa Healthcare USA, Inc; 2007. p. 379–408.

10. Bartholomew JR. Bivalirudin for the treatment of heparin-induced thrombocytopenia. In: Warkentin TE, Greinacher A, editors. Heparin-induced thrombocytopenia. 4th edition. New York: Informa Healthcare USA, Inc; 2007. p. 409–39.

11. Bradner JE, Eikelboom JW. Emerging anticoagulants and heparin-induced thrombocytopenia: indirect and direct factor Xa inhibitors and oral thrombin inhibitors. In: Warkentin TE, Greinacher A, editors. Heparin-induced thrombocytopenia. 4th edition. New York: Informa Healthcare USA, Inc; 2007. p. 441–61.

12. Warkentin TE. Heparin-induced thrombocytopenia: pathogenesis and management. Br J Haematol 2003;121(4):535–55.

13. Warkentin TE, Makris M, Jay RM, et al. A spontaneous prothrombotic disorder resembling heparin-induced thrombocytopenia. Am J Med 2008;121(7):632–6.

14. Jay RM, Warkentin TE. Fatal heparin-induced thrombocytopenia (HIT) during warfarin thromboprophylaxis following orthopedic surgery: another example of 'spontaneous' HIT? J Thromb Haemost 2008;6(9):1598–600.

15. Pruthi RK, Daniels PR, Nambudiri GS, et al. Heparin-induced thrombocytopenia (HIT) during postoperative warfarin thromboprophylaxis: a second example of postorthopedic surgery 'spontaneous' HIT? J Thromb Haemost 2009;7(3): 499–501.

16. Warkentin TE, Sheppard JI. Testing for heparin-induced thrombocytopenia antibodies. Transfus Med Rev 2006;20(4):259–72.

17. Greinacher A, Juhl D, Strobel U, et al. Heparin-induced thrombocytopenia: a prospective study on the incidence, platelet-activating capacity and clinical significance of anti-PF4/heparin antibodies of the IgG, IgM, and IgA classes. J Thromb Haemost 2007;5(8):1666–73.

18. Warkentin TE, Sheppard JI, Moore JC, et al. Quantitative interpretation of optical density measurements using PF4-dependent enzyme-immunoassays. J Thromb Haemost 2008;6(8):1304–12.

19. Warkentin TE, Kelton JG. Temporal aspects of heparin-induced thrombocytopenia. N Engl J Med 2001;344(17):1286–92.

20. Fausett MB, Vogtlander M, Lee RM, et al. Heparin-induced thrombocytopenia is rare in pregnancy. Am J Obstet Gynecol 2001;185(1):148–52.

21. Greer IA, Nelson-Piercy C. Low-molecular-weight heparins for thromboprophylaxis and treatment of venous thromboembolism in pregnancy: a systematic review of safety and efficacy. Blood 2005;106(2):401–7.

22. Warkentin TE, Sheppard JI, Siguoin CS, et al. Gender imbalance and risk factor interactions in heparin-induced thrombocytopenia. Blood 2006;108(9):2937–41.
23. Warkentin TE, Greinacher A, Koster A. Heparin-induced thrombocytopenia in patients with ventricular assist devices: are new prevention strategies required? Ann Thorac Surg 2009;87(5):1633–40.
24. Greinacher A, Alban S, Omer-Adam MA, et al. Heparin-induced thrombocytopenia: a stoichiometry-based model to explain the differing immunogenicities of unfractionated heparin, low-molecular-weight heparin, and fondaparinux in different clinical settings. Thromb Res 2008;122(2):211–20.
25. Warkentin TE, Cook RJ, Marder V, et al. Anti-PF4/heparin antibody formation post-orthopedic surgery thromboprophylaxis: the role of non-drug risk factors and evidence for a stoichiometry-based model of immunization. J Thromb Haemost 2010;8(3):504–12.
26. Lubenow N, Hinz P, Thomaschewski S, et al. The severity of trauma determines the immune response to PF4/heparin and the frequency of heparin-induced thrombocytopenia. Blood 2010;115(9):1797–803.
27. Kelton JG, Sheridan D, Santos A, et al. Heparin-induced thrombocytopenia: laboratory studies. Blood 1988;72(3):925–30.
28. Amiral J, Bridey F, Dreyfus M, et al. Platelet factor 4 complexed to heparin is the target for antibodies generated in heparin induced thrombocytopenia. Thromb Haemost 1992;68(1):95–6.
29. Greinacher A, Pötzsch B, Amiral J, et al. Heparin-associated thrombocytopenia: isolation of the antibody and characterization of a multimolecular PF4-heparin complex as the major antigen. Thromb Haemost 1994;71(2):247–51.
30. Suh JS, Aster RH, Visentin GP. Antibodies from patients with heparin-induced thrombocytopenia/thrombosis recognize different epitopes on heparin:platelet factor 4. Blood 1998;91(3):916–22.
31. Greinacher A, Gopinadhan M, Guenther JU, et al. Close approximation of two platelet factor 4 tetramers by charge neutralization forms the antigens recognized by HIT antibodies. Arterioscler Thromb Vasc Biol 2006;26(10):2386–93.
32. Warkentin TE, Levine MN, Hirsh J, et al. Heparin-induced thrombocytopenia in patients treated with low-molecular-weight heparin or unfractionated heparin. N Engl J Med 1995;332(20):1330–5.
33. Warkentin TE, Roberts RS, Hirsh J, et al. An improved definition of immune heparin-induced thrombocytopenia in postoperative orthopedic patients. Arch Intern Med 2003;163(20):2518–24.
34. Warkentin TE, Cook RJ, Marder VJ, et al. Anti-platelet factor 4/heparin antibodies in orthopedic surgery patients receiving antithrombotic prophylaxis with fondaparinux or enoxaparin. Blood 2005;106(12):3791–6.
35. Warkentin TE. An overview of the heparin-induced thrombocytopenia syndrome. Semin Thromb Hemost 2004;30(3):273–83.
36. Warkentin TE, Hayward CPM, Boshkov LK, et al. Sera from patients with heparin-induced thrombocytopenia generate platelet-derived microparticles with procoagulant activity: an explanation for the thrombotic complications of heparin-induced thrombocytopenia. Blood 1994;84(11):3691–9.
37. Arepally GM, Mayer IM. Antibodies from patients with heparin-induced thrombocytopenia stimulate monocytic cells to express tissue factor and secrete interleukin-8. Blood 2001;98(4):1252–4.
38. Warkentin TE. Clinical picture of heparin-induced thrombocytopenia. In: Warkentin TE, Greinacher A, editors. Heparin-induced thrombocytopenia. 4th edition. New York: Informa Healthcare USA, Inc; 2007. p. 21–66.

39. Greinacher A, Kohlmann T, Strobel U, et al. The temporal profile of the anti-PF4/heparin immune response. Blood 2009;113(20):4970–6.
40. Warkentin TE, Sheppard JI, Moore JC, et al. Studies of the immune response in heparin-induced thrombocytopenia. Blood 2009;113(20):4963–9.
41. Warkentin TE, Kelton JG. Delayed-onset heparin-induced thrombocytopenia and thrombosis. Ann Intern Med 2001;135(7):502–6.
42. Rice L, Attisha WK, Drexler A, et al. Delayed-onset heparin-induced thrombocytopenia. Ann Intern Med 2002;136(3):210–5.
43. Warkentin TE, Bernstein RA. Delayed-onset heparin-induced thrombocytopenia and cerebral thrombosis after a single administration of unfractionated heparin. N Engl J Med 2003;348(11):1067–9.
44. Warkentin TE. Heparin-induced thrombocytopenia: diagnosis and management. Circulation 2004;110(18):e454–8.
45. Srinivasan AF, Rice L, Bartholomew JR, et al. Warfarin-induced skin necrosis and venous limb gangrene in the setting of heparin-induced thrombocytopenia. Arch Intern Med 2004;164(1):66–70.
46. Smythe MA, Warkentin TE, Stephens JL, et al. Venous limb gangrene during overlapping therapy with warfarin and a direct thrombin inhibitor for immune heparin-induced thrombocytopenia. Am J Hematol 2002;71(1):50–2.
47. Warkentin TE. Should vitamin K be administered when HIT is diagnosed after administration of coumarin? J Thromb Haemost 2006;4(4):894–6.
48. Warkentin TE. Heparin-induced thrombocytopenia: IgG-mediated platelet activation, platelet microparticle generation, and altered procoagulant/anticoagulant balance in the pathogenesis of thrombosis and venous limb gangrene complicating heparin-induced thrombocytopenia. Transfus Med Rev 1996;10(4):249–58.
49. Warkentin TE. Venous limb gangrene during warfarin treatment of cancer-associated deep venous thrombosis. Ann Intern Med 2001;135(8 pt 1):589–93.
50. Warkentin TE. Heparin-induced thrombocytopenia. In: Colman RW, Marder VJ, Clowes AW, et al, editors. Hemostasis and thrombosis: basic principles and clinical practice. 5th edition. Philadelphia: Lippincott Williams & Wilkins; 2006. p. 1649–61.
51. Greinacher A, Warkentin TE. Treatment of heparin-induced thrombocytopenia: an overview. In: Warkentin TE, Greinacher A, editors. Heparin-induced thrombocytopenia. 4th edition. New York: Informa Healthcare USA, Inc; 2007. p. 283–317.
52. Prechel MM, McDonald MK, Jeske WP, et al. Activation of platelets by heparin-induced thrombocytopenia antibodies in the serotonin release assay is not dependent on the presence of heparin. J Thromb Haemost 2005;3(10):2168–75.
53. Socher I, Kroll H, Jorks S, et al. Heparin-independent activation of platelets by heparin-induced thrombocytopenia antibodies: a common occurrence. J Thromb Haemost 2008;6(1):197–200.
54. Newman PM, Chong BH. Heparin-induced thrombocytopenia: new evidence for the dynamic binding of purified anti-PF4-heparin antibodies to platelets and the resultant platelet activation. Blood 2000;96(1):182–7.
55. Greinacher A, Warkentin TE. The direct thrombin inhibitor hirudin. Thromb Haemost 2008;99(5):819–29.
56. Krauel K, Fürll B, Warkentin TE, et al. Heparin-induced thrombocytopenia—therapeutic concentrations of danaparoid, unlike fondaparinux and direct thrombin inhibitors, inhibit formation of PF4/heparin complexes. J Thromb Haemost 2008;6(12):2160–7.

57. Prechel M, Jeske WP, McDonald MK, et al. Desulfated heparin blocks platelet activation induced by HIT antibodies/heparin. A new approach to patient management [abstract]. Blood 2004;104(11 Pt 1 of 2):827.

58. Chong BH, Gallus AS, Cade JF, et al. Prospective randomized open-label comparison of danaparoid with dextran 70 in the treatment of heparin-induced thrombocytopenia with thrombosis: a clinical outcome study. Thromb Haemost 2001;86(5):1170–5.

59. Lubenow N, Warkentin TE, Greinacher A, et al. Results of a systematic evaluation of treatment outcomes for heparin-induced thrombocytopenia in patients receiving danaparoid, ancrod, and/or coumarin explain the rapid shift in clinical practice during the 1990s. Thromb Res 2006;117(5):507–15.

60. Farner B, Eichler P, Kroll H, et al. A comparison of danaparoid and lepirudin in heparin-induced thrombocytopenia. Thromb Haemost 2001;85(6):950–7.

61. Demers C, Ginsberg JS, Brill-Edwards P, et al. Rapid anticoagulation using ancrod for heparin-induced thrombocytopenia. Blood 1991;78(9):2194–7.

62. Warkentin TE, Maurer BT, Aster RH. Heparin-induced thrombocytopenia associated with fondaparinux. N Engl J Med 2007;356(25):2653–4.

63. Rota E, Bazzan M, Fantino G. Fondaparinux-related thrombocytopenia in a previous low-molecular-weight heparin (LMWH)-induced heparin-induced thrombocytopenia. Thromb Haemost 2008;99(4):779–81.

64. Salem M, Elrefai S, Shrit MA, et al. Fondaparinux thromboprophylaxis-associated heparin-induced thrombocytopenia syndrome complicated by catastrophic stroke. Thromb Haemost 2010, in press.

65. Kuo KHM, Kovacs MJ. Successful treatment of heparin induced thrombocytopenia (HIT) with fondaparinux. Thromb Haemost 2005;93(5):999–1000.

66. Lobo B, Finch C, Howard A, et al. Fondaparinux for the treatment of patients with acute heparin-induced thrombocytopenia. Thromb Haemost 2008;99(1):208–14.

67. Grouzi E, Kyriakou E, Panagou I, et al. Fondaparinux for the treatment of acute heparin-induced thrombocytopenia: a single-center experience. Clin Appl Thromb Hemost 2009. [Epub ahead of print].

68. Hacquard M, De Maistre E, Lecompte T. Lepirudin: is the approved dosing schedule too high? J Thromb Haemost 2005;3(11):2593–6.

69. Lubenow N, Eichler P, Lietz T, et al. Lepirudin in patients with heparin-induced thrombocytopenia—results of the third prospective study (HAT-3) and a combined analysis of HAT-1, HAT-2, and HAT-3. J Thromb Haemost 2005;3(11):2428–36.

70. Lubenow N, Eichler P, Lietz T, et al. Lepirudin for prophylaxis of thrombosis in patients with acute isolated heparin-induced thrombocytopenia: an analysis of 3 prospective studies. Blood 2004;104(10):3072–7.

71. Tardy B, Lecompte T, Boelhen F, et al. Predictive factors for thrombosis and major bleeding in an observational study in 181 patients with heparin-induced thrombocytopenia treated with lepirudin. Blood 2006;108(5):1492–6.

72. Lewis BE, Wallis DE, Berkowitz SD, et al. Argatroban anticoagulant therapy in patients with heparin-induced thrombocytopenia. Circulation 2001;103(14):1838–43.

73. Lewis BE, Wallis DE, Leya F, et al. Argatroban anticoagulation in patients with heparin-induced thrombocytopenia. Arch Intern Med 2003;163(15):1849–56.

74. Lewis BE, Wallis DE, Hursting MJ, et al. Effects of argatroban therapy, demographic variables, and platelet count on thrombotic risks in heparin-induced thrombocytopenia. Chest 2006;129(6):1407–16.

75. Warkentin TE, Greinacher A, Craven S, et al. Differences in the clinically effective molar concentrations of four direct thrombin inhibitors explain their variable prothrombin time prolongation. Thromb Haemost 2005;94(5):958–64.
76. Kaiser TH, Fish DN. Evaluation of bivalirudin treatment for heparin-induced thrombocytopenia in critically ill patients with hepatic and/or renal dysfunction. Pharmacotherapy 2006;26(4):452–60.

Heparin and Survival in Cancer Patients

Frederiek F. van Doormaal, MD*, Harry R. Büller, MD

KEYWORDS

• Cancer • Anticoagulants • Heparin

HEPARIN AND THE SURVIVAL BENEFIT IN CANCER PATIENTS: THE BIRTH OF THE HYPOTHESIS

Cancer may activate the coagulation system, which has been known since 1823 when Bouillaud[1] described three patients with cancer and venous thrombosis. In addition, cancer cells use this system specifically for their growth and metastasis. The first clinical observation of anticoagulants having an inhibitory effect on cancer growth was reported in a study published in 1992.[2] This trial compared the efficacy and safety of two types of heparin, low molecular weight heparin (LMWH) and unfractionated heparin (UFH), in the initial treatment of patients with venous thromboembolism (VTE). Unexpectedly, the subgroup of patients with VTE who also had cancer at entry had a better survival after 3 months when treated with LMWH for 5 to 10 days compared with those treated with UFH.

A meta-analysis published in 1998 of all VTE treatment studies confirmed this finding. In patients with VTE who had cancer, the observed 3-month mortality rate was 15.0% (46/306) for those initially treated with LMWH compared with 22.0% (71/323) in those who received UFH during the initial treatment period for their VTE (odds ratio, 0.61; 95% CI, 0.40–0.93). In contrast, among patients with VTE who did not have cancer (odds ratio, 0.94; 95% CI, 0.60–1.47), the 3-month mortality rate was 2.6% (39/1481) for those in the LMWH group versus 2.8% (41/1471) for those in the UFH group.[3]

Adjustment for the primary site of the cancer, age, and gender was performed among data from 3 trials involving 1921 patients, of whom 405 had cancer. In patients with VTE who had cancer, the odds ratio was 0.62 (95% CI 0.36–1.08) for those treated with LMWH, whereas no differences in thrombotic or bleeding complications were noted between those treated with LMWH and those treated with UFH.[4]

Further adjustment for histology, tumour stage, sites of metastases, duration of cancer, and cancer treatment could be made in one trial with 1021 patients, in which 198 patients with cancer had been included. Of the 103 patients with cancer who were

Department of Vascular Medicine, Academic Medical Center Amsterdam, Meibergdreef 9, 1105 AZ Amsterdam, Netherlands
* Corresponding author.
E-mail address: F.F.vanDoormaal@amc.uva.nl

Hematol Oncol Clin N Am 24 (2010) 777–784
doi:10.1016/j.hoc.2010.05.003
0889-8588/10/$ – see front matter © 2010 Elsevier Inc. All rights reserved.

hemonc.theclinics.com

treated with LMWH, 19 died within 3 months after study entry, compared with 25 of 95 patients who had cancer in the UFH arm. Without correction for these prognostic factors, the odds ratio was 0.63 (95% CI, 0.32–1.24). After adjusting for histology (adenocarcinoma), stage of the disease (TNM), metastases and site of the tumour, duration of the disease (<1 year; 1–2 years), and treatment, the odds ratio became 0.39 (95% CI, 0.15–1.02), indicating that these adjustments did not change the originally observed beneficial effects of LMWH.[4]

Of course these analyses have several limitations. First, they concern studies with another objective, which was treatment of acute venous thrombotic disease, and the follow-up period was usually limited to 3 months. Second, only patients with cancer who had symptomatic VTE were included, and therefore the relevance for those without VTE remained uncertain. Furthermore, two heparins were compared and therefore the benefit of LMWH alone is unclear. Finally, the types of malignancies varied widely. Nevertheless, the effects were so impressive that randomized controlled trials of the effect of LMWH on cancer progression in patients without VTE were subsequently initiated.

HEPARIN IN PATIENTS WITH CANCER WITHOUT VTE

Six clinical trials have been published studying heparin in patients with cancer without VTE. The inhibitory effects of heparin on cancer growth were studied for the first time in a randomized controlled trial published in 1994, in which 277 patients with both limited and extensive small cell lung cancer were included.[5] Patients were randomized to receive either a prophylactic dose of UFH for 5 weeks or no heparin in addition to their chemotherapy. The response rate was 37% in patients receiving UFH compared with 23% in those receiving only chemotherapy ($P = .004$). The median survival time was 317 days in the UFH group compared with 261 days in the no-UFH group ($P = .01$). During long-term follow-up (ie, 1, 2, and 3 years after study entry), the survival rates were better in patients receiving UFH, which was statistically significant for those with limited small cell lung cancer.

Altinbas and colleagues[6] also randomized 84 patients with both limited and extensive small cell lung cancer to either a prophylactic dose of a LMWH (dalteparin) or placebo in combination with chemotherapy for a maximum of 18 weeks. The response rate was 69.2% in the patients treated with LMWH, with an overall median survival of 13.0 months, versus 42.5% and 8.0 months, respectively, in the no-LMWH group ($P = .07$ and $P = .01$, respectively).

The FAMOUS trial included a heterogeneous group of 385 patients,[7] all of whom had advanced disease (stage III or IV) and a minimum life expectancy of 3 months. Patients were randomized to receive either a prophylactic dose of a LMWH (dalteparin) or placebo for 12 months with no restriction on concomitant chemotherapy or radiotherapy. At 1, 2, and 3 years, a trend for a better survival was observed in the LMWH group; however, this was significant in a post-hoc analysis in patients who were alive at 17 months after study entry.

A subgroup of patients with cancer who had better survival at study entry (>6 months) was predefined in the MALT study published in 2006.[8] In this randomized trial, 302 patients with different types of advanced cancer that could not be treated curatively and who had a minimum life expectancy of 1 month were randomized to receive either a LMWH (nadroparin; 2 weeks therapeutic dose followed by 4 weeks of a prophylactic dose) or placebo for 6 weeks. The overall median survival was 8.0 months in the nadroparin recipients versus 6.6 months in the placebo group (overall hazard ratio [HR], 0.75; 95% CI, 0.59–0.96). However, in the subgroup of patients with limited disease, defined as an expected survival of at least 6 months at the start, the median survival was 15.4 months versus 9.4 months in the LMWH group and the placebo group, respectively (HR, 0.64; 95% CI, 0.45–0.90).

Sideras and colleagues[9] recruited 141 patients with different types of advanced cancer, a minimum life expectancy of 12 weeks, and an Eastern Cooperative Oncology Group performance status of 0 to 2 to either a prophylactic dose of a LMWH (dalteparin) or placebo or no intervention. The duration of heparin treatment is unclear, but study outcomes included mortality at 1, 2, and 3 years. However, no clinically or statistically significant effect was shown.

In the most recent published study among 69 patients with advanced pancreatic cancer, Icli and colleagues[10] combined LMWH with standard anticancer treatment in 35 patients. Although a clear survival benefit was observed for those treated with LMWH, this study was not randomized and therefore these results should be interpreted with caution.

WHAT IS THE RELATIONSHIP BETWEEN CANCER AND THE ACTIVATION OF HEMOSTASIS?

Cancer cells can express several coagulation proteins, thereby activating the coagulation system at several levels. Tissue factor, the initiator of the coagulation system, is expressed by several cancer types.[11–13] Furthermore, chemokines, such as tumour necrosis factor α, are excreted by cancer cells and can activate monocytes and macrophages, resulting in tissue factor expression on these cells.[14] Lower levels of activated protein C, a natural anticoagulant protein, are observed in patients with cancer because of down-regulation of thrombomodulin on the endothelial cells by these released chemokines, thereby further contributing to the hypercoagulable state.[15] In addition, cancer cells can express urokinase-type and tissue-type plasminogen activators, plasminogen-activator inhibitor 1 and 2, and the plasminogen-activator receptor. The balance among these fibrinolytic proteins leads to an impaired fibrinolysis.[16]

A more recent factor contributing to the hypercoagulable state in patients with cancer is circulating microparticles. Different types of cells, including cancer cells and platelets, are able to form these cell membrane–derived particles. Their phospholipid membrane can bind several coagulation factors. Particles derived from activated monocytes and endothelial and cancer cells can express tissue factor, making them procoagulant. In patients with cancer, high levels of these microparticles have been associated with the occurrence of venous thrombosis and a worse prognosis.[17,18]

The formation of the end product of the coagulation system, fibrin, around the cancer cells supports angiogenesis and protects the cancer cells against immune attacks.[19]

Furthermore, individual coagulation proteins, irrespective of their role in fibrin formation, create a favorable environment for cancer growth. Binding of FVIIa to the extracellular domain of tissue factor increases the amount of intracellular calcium. This increase activates protein kinase C, which in turn phosphorylates the cytoplasmic tail of tissue factor, which subsequently enhances cancer cell motility and migration and the production of growth factors.[20]

Thrombin stimulates the expression of adhesion molecules on cancer cells and the production of chemokines through binding to protein activated receptors (PARs), members of the G-coupled receptors. Four PAR receptors have been described. PAR signalling increases cancer cell motility and survival and the production of growth factors. Thrombin mainly binds to PAR-1 and PAR-4, whereas other coagulation factors, such as the TF-FVIIa complex and FXa, can activate PAR-2. Furthermore, thrombin activates platelets by binding to their PAR-1 receptor.[20] The activated platelets express P-selectin, a ligand for the adhesion of cancer cells. A shield of platelets is formed and protects cancer cells in the bloodstream from the immune system.

The expression of adhesion molecules on endothelial cells is upregulated by thrombin. Adhesion of cancer cells to the activated platelets and the endothelium facilitates extravasation.[21] Finally, large amounts of growth factors are released by activated platelets, especially vascular endothelial growth factor. In addition to its well-known angiogenic stimulating properties, this hormone causes leakage of plasma proteins through the vessel wall, including fibrinogen, creating again a proangiogenic environment.[19]

IS THERE FUNDAMENTAL EVIDENCE FOR THE CLINICAL OBSERVATIONS OF THE EFFECT OF LMWH?

The proposed mechanisms of the suppressive effects of heparin on cancer progression are mainly based on in vitro and in vivo studies. Heparins impair cancer growth and progression through several possible mechanisms: decrease of thrombin and fibrin formation; binding to adhesion molecules; anti-heparanase effects; and increase of apoptosis.

Heparins have well-known anticoagulant effects resulting in inhibition of thrombin and fibrin formation. Thrombin and fibrin are important for cancer growth and progression. In addition to its anticoagulant effects, heparin is thought to have other properties, illustrated by the antimetastatic effects of nonanticoagulant heparins.[22]

The first nonanticoagulant mechanism of heparin is interference with the interaction between cancer cells and platelets. Specific oligosaccharide structures in heparin can bind to P-selectins exposed on activated platelets[23]; these structures show minimal anticoagulant activity. Ludwig and colleagues[24] tested the impact of UFH, LMWH (nadroparin and enoxaparin), and fondaparinux on P-selectin–dependent tumor interactions in vitro and metastasis formation in vivo. These agents differ widely in their potential to interfere with P-selectin–mediated cell binding. This inhibitory function strongly correlates to the potency in inhibiting experimental lung metastasis in vivo.[25]

Selectins are also expressed on leukocytes (L-selectin) and the vascular endothelium (E- and P-selectin). Heparin can inhibit L-selectin binding to its ligands, resulting in inhibition of the inflammatory response. Furthermore, extravasation of cancer cells is hindered by binding of heparin to selectins.[23,26,27]

The second nonanticoagulant property of heparin is inhibition of cancer cell heparanase,[28] which is expressed in many human cancers. This enzyme breaks down the polysaccharide barrier, facilitating cancer cell invasion through the vascular basement membrane and promoting angiogenesis and metastases.[29] In humans, elevated heparanase expression by tumors has been correlated with more aggressive behavior in breast, colon, ovary, pancreas, and non-small lung cancers, and acute myeloid leukemia and myeloma tumors.[30–37] Heparanase also cleaves the growth factors bearing heparan sulphate groups from heparan sulphate proteogylcans localized in the extracellular matrix and cellular membranes.[38–40] Heparins can also directly inhibit the effect of growth factors. LMWH hinders binding of growth factors to high-affinity receptors to a greater degree than UFH.[41]

Heparin, especially LMWH, is thought to increase the apoptosis index in cancer cells. Nasir and colleagues[42] observed a fourfold increase in the apoptosis index in heparin knockout mice given LMWH compared with controls. Heparin probably enters the cell through endocytosis and induces apoptosis by interfering with transcription factor.[43]

LATEST RESULTS

The preliminary results of the latest clinical trial (INPACT) on the effect of LMWH on cancer growth were presented at the XXII International Society on Thrombosis and Haemostasis (ISTH) Congress 2009. This multicenter, randomized, open-label study was performed in patients with either non-small cell lung cancer (stage IIIB) within 3 months after diagnosis, hormone refractory prostate cancer within 6 months after diagnosis, or locally advanced pancreatic cancer within 3 months after diagnosis. Patients were randomized to nadroparin, a LMWH, or no nadroparin in addition to their standard anticancer treatment. Subcutaneous nadroparin was given at therapeutic doses for 2 weeks, followed by half therapeutic doses for 4 weeks. Patients were subsequently eligible for six cycles of 2-week periods of nadroparin at therapeutic doses at every 6 weeks. The minimum duration of follow-up was 46 weeks.

Outcomes were overall survival and major bleeding. All study outcomes were adjudicated by an independent and blinded committee. A total of 503 patients were included between May 2006 and August 2008. Of these, 244 patients received nadroparin and 259 were allocated to no nadroparin. The intention-to-treat population consisted of 197 patients with prostate cancer, 170 with non-small cell lung cancer, and 135 with pancreatic cancer.

At the preliminary analysis in July 2009, the overall mortality was 55.7% (n = 136) in the nadroparin arm compared with 62.2% (n = 161) in the no-treatment group (HR, 0.92; 95% CI, 0.73–1.16). The median survival was 12.5 months in the nadroparin recipients and 11.9 months in the no-treatment subjects. Survival analysis in the three cancer types separately also did not show a statistically significant difference between the groups; however, a trend for better survival in patients with prostate cancer was observed (HR, 0.77; 95% CI, 0.52–1.15). The proportion of patients having at least one episode of major bleeding was comparable, with 4.1% in the nadroparin recipients (n = 10) and 3.5% in the no-treatment arm (n = 9).

Summary of the Results

In contrast to the survival benefit shown in the studies mentioned earlier, the preliminary result of the latest and largest trial did not show a statistically or clinically significant effect. The earlier MALT study was the foundation for the INPACT study and a comparable treatment strategy was applied. How can these negative results of the study be explained? In the MALT study the effect was more significant in the patients with limited disease at baseline; their survival was 9.4 months in the placebo group compared with 15.4 months in group treated with nadroparin. Therefore, patient groups with a comparable prognosis were selected for the INPACT study. The selection of the patients seemed to be successful, with a comparable median survival of 11.9 months in the control group. Second, the successful treatment strategy, consisting of 2 weeks therapeutic dose followed by half that dose for 4 weeks, was used initially. Moreover, patients were encouraged to receive a maximum of six repeated cycles of nadroparin at therapeutic dose. The latter strategy was based on the hypothesis that repetitive exposure to LMWH may increase the effect, and intended to try to circumvent adaptive processes in the cancer cells when LMWH should be administered continuously for a prolonged period. It is unlikely, but not impossible, that the repeated courses may have diminished the anticancer effect. Finally, the study had sufficient power to detect a clinically and significantly important difference in survival between the groups.

How do the preliminary results of the INPACT trial impact on the overall assessment of LMWH? **Fig. 1** shows a previously unpublished meta-analysis of all randomised

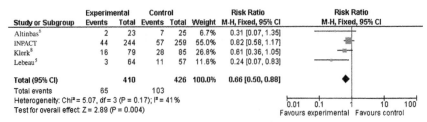

Fig. 1. Mortality in cancer patients without VTE with a prognosis of at least six months at study entry.

controlled trials that selected a patient group with limited disease.[5,6,8] In total, 410 patients with limited-stage cancer at study entry were treated with heparin, compared with 426 patients treated with placebo or who did not receive treatment. In the heparin group, 16% of the patients (65/410) died during the study period compared with 24% of the control subjects (103/426), resulting in an HR of 0.66 (95% CI, 0.50–0.88) for overall survival after 6 months favoring heparin treatment.

PRACTICAL ADVICE

The clinical evidence for a survival benefit associated with LMWH for patients who have cancer without VTE is still not convincing. Therefore, patients who have cancer without VTE should not be routinely treated with LMWH. However, further research is justified to unravel the potential anticancer mechanisms of the heparin molecule. Furthermore, ongoing trials on the survival effect of LMWH should be awaited. The effect of LMWH does not seem to be cancer type–specific. Therefore, a small anti-cancer effect per patient would result in a large overall survival benefit. Aside from the well-known bleeding risk, LMWH treatment has no other important side effects. Moreover, it lowers the risk for VTE in a population with a 10% risk of developing this condition.

REFERENCES

1. Bouillaud. De L'Obliteration des veines et de son influence sur la formation des hydropisies partielles: considerations sur la hydropisies passives en general. Archives generales de medicine 1823;1:188–204.
2. Prandoni P, Lensing AW, Buller HR, et al. Comparison of subcutaneous low-molecular-weight heparin with intravenous standard heparin in proximal deep-vein thrombosis. Lancet 1992;339(8791):441–5.
3. Hettiarachchi RJ, Prins MH, Lensing AW, et al. Low molecular weight heparin versus unfractionated heparin in the initial treatment of venous thromboembolism. Curr Opin Pulm Med 1998;4(4):220–5.
4. Hettiarachchi RJ, Smorenburg SM, Ginsberg J, et al. Do heparins do more than just treat thrombosis? The influence of heparins on cancer spread. Thromb Haemost 1999;82(2):947–52.
5. Lebeau B, Chastang C, Brechot JM, et al. Subcutaneous heparin treatment increases survival in small cell lung cancer. "Petites Cellules" Group. Cancer 1994;74(1):38–45.
6. Altinbas M, Coskun HS, Er O, et al. A randomized clinical trial of combination chemotherapy with and without low-molecular-weight heparin in small cell lung cancer. J Thromb Haemost 2004;2(8):1266–71.

7. Kakkar AK, Levine MN, Kadziola Z, et al. Low molecular weight heparin, therapy with dalteparin, and survival in advanced cancer: the fragmin advanced malignancy outcome study (FAMOUS). J Clin Oncol 2004;22(10):1944–8.
8. Klerk CP, Smorenburg SM, Otten HM, et al. The effect of low molecular weight heparin on survival in patients with advanced malignancy. J Clin Oncol 2005; 23(10):2130–5.
9. Sideras K, Schaefer PL, Okuno SH, et al. Low-molecular-weight heparin in patients with advanced cancer: a phase 3 clinical trial. Mayo Clin Proc 2006; 81(6):758–67.
10. Icli F, Akbulut H, Utkan G, et al. Low molecular weight heparin (LMWH) increases the efficacy of cisplatinum plus gemcitabine combination in advanced pancreatic cancer. J Surg Oncol 2007;95(6):507–12.
11. Haas SL, Jesnowski R, Steiner M, et al. Expression of tissue factor in pancreatic adenocarcinoma is associated with activation of coagulation. World J Gastroenterol 2006;12(30):4843–9.
12. Uno K, Homma S, Satoh T, et al. Tissue factor expression as a possible determinant of thromboembolism in ovarian cancer. Br J Cancer 2007;96(2):290–5.
13. Yamashita H, Kitayama J, Ishikawa M, et al. Tissue factor expression is a clinical indicator of lymphatic metastasis and poor prognosis in gastric cancer with intestinal phenotype. J Surg Oncol 2007;95(4):324–31.
14. Rickles FR, Hair GA, Zeff RA, et al. Tissue factor expression in human leukocytes and tumor cells. Thromb Haemost 1995;74(1):391–5.
15. Hanly AM, Winter DC. The role of thrombomodulin in malignancy. Semin Thromb Hemost 2007;33(7):673–9.
16. McMahon B, Kwaan HC. The plasminogen activator system and cancer. Pathophysiol Haemost Thromb 2008;36(3–4):184–94.
17. Furie B, Furie BC. Mechanisms of thrombus formation. N Engl J Med 2008;359(9): 938–49.
18. Tesselaar ME, Romijn FP, van dL I, et al. Microparticle-associated tissue factor activity: a link between cancer and thrombosis? J Thromb Haemost 2007;5(3): 520–7.
19. Rickles FR, Patierno S, Fernandez PM. Tissue factor, thrombin, and cancer. Chest 2003;124(Suppl 3):58S–68S.
20. Ruf W, Mueller BM. Thrombin generation and the pathogenesis of cancer. Semin Thromb Hemost 2006;32(Suppl):161–8.
21. Borsig L. The role of platelet activation in tumor metastasis. Expert Rev Anticancer Ther 2008;8(8):1247–55.
22. Kragh M, Loechel F. Non-anti-coagulant heparins: a promising approach for prevention of tumor metastasis [review]. Int J Oncol 2005;27(4):1159–67.
23. Wang L, Brown JR, Varki A, et al. Heparin's anti-inflammatory effects require glucosamine 6-O-sulfation and are mediated by blockade of L- and P-selectins. J Clin Invest 2002;110(1):127–36.
24. Ludwig RJ, Alban S, Bistrian R, et al. The ability of different forms of heparins to suppress P-selectin function in vitro correlates to their inhibitory capacity on bloodborne metastasis in vivo. Thromb Haemost 2006;95(3):535–40.
25. Stevenson JL, Choi SH, Varki A. Differential metastasis inhibition by clinically relevant levels of heparins–correlation with selectin inhibition, not antithrombotic activity. Clin Cancer Res 2005;11(19 Pt 1):7003–11.
26. Varki NM, Varki A. Heparin inhibition of selectin-mediated interactions during the hematogenous phase of carcinoma metastasis: rationale for clinical studies in humans. Semin Thromb Hemost 2002;28(1):53–66.

27. Nelson RM, Cecconi O, Roberts WG, et al. Heparin oligosaccharides bind L- and P-selectin and inhibit acute inflammation. Blood 1993;82(11):3253–8.

28. Parish CR, Freeman C, Brown KJ, et al. Identification of sulfated oligosaccharide-based inhibitors of tumor growth and metastasis using novel in vitro assays for angiogenesis and heparanase activity. Cancer Res 1999;59(14):3433–41.

29. Vlodavsky I, Friedmann Y, Elkin M, et al. Mammalian heparanase: gene cloning, expression and function in tumor progression and metastasis. Nat Med 1999; 5(7):793–802.

30. Maxhimer JB, Quiros RM, Stewart R, et al. Heparanase-1 expression is associated with the metastatic potential of breast cancer. Surgery 2002;132(2):326–33.

31. Friedmann Y, Vlodavsky I, Aingorn H, et al. Expression of heparanase in normal, dysplastic, and neoplastic human colonic mucosa and stroma. Evidence for its role in colonic tumorigenesis. Am J Pathol 2000;157(4):1167–75.

32. Ginath S, Menczer J, Friedmann Y, et al. Expression of heparanase, Mdm2, and erbB2 in ovarian cancer. Int J Oncol 2001;18(6):1133–44.

33. Gohji K, Okamoto M, Kitazawa S, et al. Heparanase protein and gene expression in bladder cancer. J Urol 2001;166(4):1286–90.

34. Koliopanos A, Friess H, Kleeff J, et al. Heparanase expression in primary and metastatic pancreatic cancer. Cancer Res 2001;61(12):4655–9.

35. Bitan M, Polliack A, Zecchina G, et al. Heparanase expression in human leukemias is restricted to acute myeloid leukemias. Exp Hematol 2002;30(1):34–41.

36. Takahashi H, Ebihara S, Okazaki T, et al. Clinical significance of heparanase activity in primary resected non-small cell lung cancer. Lung Cancer 2004; 45(2):207–14.

37. Yang Y, Macleod V, Bendre M, et al. Heparanase promotes the spontaneous metastasis of myeloma cells to bone. Blood 2005;105(3):1303–9.

38. Ishai-Michaeli R, Eldor A, Vlodavsky I. Heparanase activity expressed by platelets, neutrophils, and lymphoma cells releases active fibroblast growth factor from extracellular matrix. Cell Regul 1990;1(11):833–42.

39. Whitelock JM, Murdoch AD, Iozzo RV, et al. The degradation of human endothelial cell-derived perlecan and release of bound basic fibroblast growth factor by stromelysin, collagenase, plasmin, and heparanases. J Biol Chem 1996;271(17): 10079–86.

40. Sanderson RD, Yang Y, Suva LJ, et al. Heparan sulfate proteoglycans and heparanase–partners in osteolytic tumor growth and metastasis. Matrix Biol 2004; 23(6):341–52.

41. Jayson GC, Gallagher JT. Heparin oligosaccharides: inhibitors of the biological activity of bFGF on Caco-2 cells. Br J Cancer 1997;75(1):9–16.

42. Nasir FA, Patel HK, Scully MF, et al. The low molecular weight heparins dalteparin sodium inhibits angiogenesis and induces apoptosis in an experimental tumour model [abstract]. Blood 2003;102(11):808.

43. Linhardt RJ. Heparin-induced cancer cell death. Chem Biol 2004;11(4):420–2.

Index

Note: Page numbers of article titles are in **boldface** type.

Hematol Oncol Clin N Am 24 (2010) 785–791
doi:10.1016/S0889-8588(10)00108-5
0889-8588/10/$ – see front matter © 2010 Elsevier Inc. All rights reserved.

hemonc.theclinics.com

Moving?

Make sure your subscription moves with you!

To notify us of your new address, find your **Clinics Account Number** (located on your mailing label above your name), and contact customer service at:

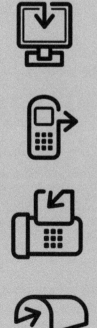

Email: journalscustomerservice-usa@elsevier.com

800-654-2452 (subscribers in the U.S. & Canada)
314-447-8871 (subscribers outside of the U.S. & Canada)

Fax number: 314-447-8029

Elsevier Health Sciences Division
Subscription Customer Service
3251 Riverport Lane
Maryland Heights, MO 63043

*To ensure uninterrupted delivery of your subscription, please notify us at least 4 weeks in advance of move.

Printed and bound by CPI Group (UK) Ltd, Croydon, CR0 4YY

03/10/2024

01040447-0012